Albert F. (Albert Franklin) Blaisdell

How to Keep Well

A Text Book of Health

Albert F. (Albert Franklin) Blaisdell

How to Keep Well
A Text Book of Health

ISBN/EAN: 9783744650052

Printed in Europe, USA, Canada, Australia, Japan

Cover: Foto ©Andreas Hilbeck / pixelio.de

More available books at **www.hansebooks.com**

HOW TO KEEP WELL

A TEXT-BOOK OF HEALTH FOR USE IN THE LOWER GRADE OF
SCHOOLS WITH SPECIAL REFERENCE TO THE EFFECTS
OF ALCOHOLIC DRINKS, TOBACCO AND
OTHER NARCOTICS ON THE
BODILY LIFE

BY

ALBERT F. BLAISDELL, M.D.

AUTHOR OF "OUR BODIES, AND HOW WE LIVE," "CHILD'S BOOK
OF HEALTH," ETC., ETC.

REVISED EDITION

BOSTON, U.S.A.
GINN & COMPANY, PUBLISHERS
1893

The Athenæum Press
GINN & COMPANY, BOSTON, U.S.A

PREFACE

THE author has aimed in this little book to present clearly and tersely the simplest facts concerning our bodily life.

Physiology is of little value to pupils in the lower grade of schools merely as a scientific study : it is of interest only so far as it treats in an attractive style of simple matters of every-day health. Yet, to understand even the plainest rules of health, we need to know something about the structure and use of the various parts of "the house we live in."

To this end, a few facts about anatomy and physiology have been presented in each chapter. To make the book more attractive and interesting, the author has used a familiar style, weaving into the text such incidental matter as will serve to arouse the interest and rivet the attention of the young pupil.

The real object of studying physiology in our schools is to teach young folks how to keep well and strong ; and to avoid evil habits that destroy character as well as health. Hence special emphasis has been laid upon such points as have a practical bearing upon the personal care of health.

Special reference has been made to the nature and effect

iii

of alcoholic drinks, tobacco, and other narcotics upon the human system. Such facts concerning their physiological action have been discussed as can be easily understood by those for whom these pages have been written.

This book has been thoroughly revised. A new chapter on the subject of alcoholic drinks and other narcotics has been added, together with much additional material on the same subject.

The new chapter on Practical Experiments will commend itself both to the teacher and the pupil. Nothing can take the place of a systematic series of practical experiments in teaching physiology, even with the youngest class of boys and girls.

In the preparation of this revised and enlarged edition, the author and publishers are under deep obligations to Mrs. Mary H. Hunt, the Superintendent of the Department of Scientific Instruction of the National Woman's Christian Temperance Union, who has carefully revised the work.

ALBERT F. BLAISDELL.

PROVIDENCE, R.I., November 1891.

CONTENTS

𝕭𝖑𝖆𝖎𝖘𝖉𝖊𝖑𝖑'𝖘 𝕽𝖊𝖛𝖎𝖘𝖊𝖉 𝕾𝖊𝖗𝖎𝖊𝖘 𝖔𝖋 𝕻𝖍𝖞𝖘𝖎𝖔𝖑𝖔𝖌𝖎𝖊𝖘

FOR ADVANCED SCHOOLS

YOUNG FOLKS' PHYSIOLOGY
A REVISED EDITION OF
"OUR BODIES AND HOW WE LIVE"

An elementary treatise on Physiology and Hygiene for families and schools, with especial reference to the effects of alcoholic drinks, tobacco, and other narcotics on the human system. *Illustrated.*

FOR LOWER SCHOOLS

PHYSIOLOGY FOR BOYS AND GIRLS
A REVISED EDITION OF
"HOW TO KEEP WELL"

A text-book of health for use in the lower grades of schools, with special reference to the effects of alcoholic drinks, tobacco, and other narcotics on the bodily life. *Illustrated.*

FOR PRIMARY SCHOOLS

PHYSIOLOGY FOR LITTLE FOLKS
A REVISED EDITION OF
"THE CHILD'S BOOK OF HEALTH".

In easy lessons for younger scholars. *Illustrated.*

INDORSEMENT

This series of books having been revised under our advice and supervision, and containing a full and fair treatment of the nature and effects of alcoholic drinks, tobacco, and other narcotics, in connection with relative Physiology and Hygiene, expressed in language which pupils — in the grades for which the books are intended — can readily comprehend, we take great pleasure in recommending the same for use as SCHOOL TEXT-BOOKS.

ADVISORY BOARD

Albert H. Plumb, D.D.

Daniel Dorchester, D.D.

Hon. William E. Sheldon.

Rev. Joseph Cook.

MARY H. HUNT

National and International Superintendent Department of Scientific Instruction of the Woman's Christian Temperance Union. Life Director of National Educational Association.

DECEMBER 5, 1891.

HOW TO KEEP WELL

CHAPTER I

INTRODUCTION

1. What the Book is about. — When we get used to any common event, as, for example, to seeing a boy or girl moving, talking, and breathing, we forget to wonder at it, simply because it is so common a sight. But, when one does think about it, how very wonderful it is to be alive !

One begins to ask, How do we manage to move our bodies ? When one has hurt his foot, how does his head know that he has done so ? Why do we breathe and eat ? How do we think ? and how do we speak ?

All these things this little book will try to explain to you. There will not be room to tell you about all the wonders of our bodies, but you will be able to learn the beginning of the story. There is much more to learn. When you have learned all that is told you here, you will feel so much interested, we hope, that you will wish to learn more.

The study of our bodies will not only make us acquainted with many wonderful things, but will also tell us how to get good health and how to keep it.

Therefore let us do our best to learn as much as possible about our bodies, and how we live.

2. Our Bodily Life. — We need not be told that our bodies are made of flesh and bone, whose substance we see and handle every day of our lives. Even a child knows that certain parts of his body, as the walls of his chest, and his heart that he feels beating within it, are always moving of themselves.

We can move of our own free will from one place to another. The wind may rustle the leaves, and a breeze may sway a strong oak; but the leaves and the oak have no power to move themselves. We need not wait, like the trees of the forest, for the wind to blow us to and fro, or, like the pebbles by the roadside, for some one to stir us. Like the horse, the dog, the bird, or any other animal that has life, we can move from place to place.

Again: every child cannot but notice that he is always warm. Even in the coldest day of midwinter, let the stones and trees be as cold as the winter wind, our bodies, except perhaps the tips of the fingers and toes, are always warm. The horse, the dog, and even the birds and the bees, are warm; all animals, in fact, are more or less warm as long as they are alive.

3. The Body compared to a Steam-Engine. — Our bodies are in some ways very much like a steam-engine. The bones and the muscles resemble the machinery of the engine, while the motive-power is produced by the food we eat.

We put fuel into the furnace. The water in the boiler is heated, and expands into steam. Then the piston-rod begins to work to and fro : this moves the wheels, joints, and levers, and so the whole engine is set in motion by the fuel in the furnace.

Now, just the same thing occurs in our bodies. We take food, and that food passes into the stomach and is changed into blood. By reason of that food we are kept warm, strength is developed, and the levers and joints within us are set working, as we see in the steam-engine.

There is, however, this important difference between the two : The engine is all the time wearing itself out : it works badly now and then, so it must be stopped, taken to pieces, and repaired.

Our bodies, too, are all the time wearing out ; but they are continually repairing themselves, even while in constant use. Hence we take food, not only to warm us, but also to build up and repair our bodies.

4. **The Body and its Nervous System.** — Every child knows that when he cuts his finger with a knife, touches a hot stove, or has eaten unwholesome food, as an unripe apple, pain is produced. Silvery-white cords, called nerves, start from the brain, and are spread all over the body ; and, when anything wrong happens, these little nerves, like telegraph-wires, carry special despatches to the central station (that is, to the brain), and thus the feeling of pain is there made known. In this way every part of our bodies is watched over and protected.

If it were not so, we should be continually hurting ourselves, and not know it. For example, a drunken man, whose nerves had been deadened by alcoholic liquors, once went to sleep by a camp-fire ; and, when he woke up, his feet were so horribly burned that they had to be cut off. If his brain and nerves had not been benumbed, he would have felt the alarm of pain and saved himself.

If we exert our will, or "make up our mind," as we call it, to write with a pen, to pick a flower, or to call the name of some friend, we can do it. The mind, or brain, wills to do this or that thing. It sends out its order by the tiny white nerves, and the muscles are put in motion to do whatever the brain has willed them to do. This mind, which feels and thinks, but which we cannot see, forms the real part of our being. It is the power to feel, to know, to reason, and to will, that makes us what we are.

When we stop to think about it, how wonderful it is ! Indeed, the more we think of it, the more we shall realize the fact that the all-wise Creator, in his goodness and wisdom, has given us bodies which, in the words of the Psalmist, are "fearfully and wonderfully made."

5. **Some Hard Words explained.** — Before we can reach the more interesting part of our study, we have to do something like cracking the shell of a nut to get at its kernel : we shall have to learn the meaning of a few hard words which must be used in talking about this subject, and will be often used in this book.

Before we can tell how plants and animals *live*, we must know what plants and animals *are*. A watchmaker could not describe the working of a watch unless he first carefully learned the various parts. So it is with the study of our bodies : we must learn their structure before we can understand the manner in which they act and move, or, in short, how they live.

The science which tells us about the structure, form, and position of the different parts of our bodies, is called **Anatomy.** It tells us what these parts are, where they are, and how they look.

The science which explains the uses of the different parts of the body is called **Physiology.**

Now, after we have learned something about the structure and the uses of different parts of the body, we ought to learn how to take care of them and to keep them in health.

We do this by the study of **Hygiene,** or the science which tells us about health.

Take the skin for an illustration. If we learn what it is, how it looks, its various parts, this would be its Anatomy. Now, if we learn for what special purpose it is made, just what its different parts do, and how they do it, this would be its Physiology. Finally, if we learn how each part is kept in good order, what will injure its health, and what will do it good, this would be its Hygiene.

A **tissue** is the simplest form in which any part of the body can exist.

We thus speak of the skin as a tissue, bony tissue, muscular tissue, fatty tissue, and so on. Each tissue has certain features about it which mark it wherever in the body it is found. They may be compared to the brick, stone, iron, mortar, glass, and other materials which, properly arranged, make up a house.

Any part of the body which does a special work is called an **organ.**

It is simply several tissues working together as a whole, and specially fitted to do a certain thing : thus the eye is the organ of sight, the nose of smell, the ear of hearing, the stomach of digestion, and so on.

When there is a series of organs scattered through the body, similar in structure, and all doing the same work, we call it a "system:" thus we speak of the arterial system, the nervous system, and so on.

The special work which an organ has to do is said to be the **function,** or use, of that organ : thus it is the function of the eye to see, and of the stomach to digest food.   The word "glands" will be often used.

Glands are curious organs, of various shapes and sizes, whose special work it is to make out of the blood something to be used again, or to rid the blood of something to be cast out of the body.   Thus the salivary glands make saliva, or spittle, and the sweat glands make sweat.   The liver, which weighs about five pounds, is a single gland, and secretes bile ; while the glands in the intestines cannot be seen by the naked eye.

6. General Parts of the Body. — If we look at our body, we see that it is made up of a middle, barrel-shaped part, called the **trunk.**   Above this is placed a kind of round ball, called the **head;** while two pairs of branches, called the **limbs,** are attached to the upper and lower corners of the trunk.

Again, we see that the whole body has an outer covering, the *skin.*   Underneath the skin lie long bundles of red flesh, called *muscles.*   These are mostly fastened at each end to the hard parts or bones.

The bones make up the framework or **skeleton** of our bodies.

The limbs are solid, but the head is hollow, and holds an organ called the *brain*, the centre of the nervous system. A cheesy-like substance, called the *spinal cord*, passes from the brain down the middle of the backbone, and sends its thread-like branches, called *nerves*, all over the body. It is through the nervous system that we are able to think or feel, or, in fact, to know anything.

Most of the organs of the body are in the **trunk.** Suppose we take away the skin, the muscles, and the ribs, which hide the inside of the body from us, and what shall we see? Perhaps you have wondered how your heart, your lungs, and all the other parts which you know you have in your body, are arranged.

You may be able to see, very likely, the body of some dead animal, such as a rabbit or a pig, cut open. If you can, this will give you a better idea of your own self than any picture can do. The inside of our body is very nearly like that of one of the lower animals. They have the same organs we have, doing the same work. If you can see the inside of any animal, you will be sure to notice how closely and carefully the organs are packed in the **trunk.** There is no space for any one of them to move about; if one ever is pushed from its place, it must crowd upon and hurt another.

One of the first things you will notice in Figs. 1 and 2 is a partition, in the form of an arch, separating

the top part of the trunk from the bottom. This is
called the *diaphragm*.

It makes the trunk a two-story house, — the abdomen
down-stairs, and the heart and lungs in the chamber.
Above the diaphragm — that is, in the chamber, or
chest [thorax] — are the heart
and the two lungs.

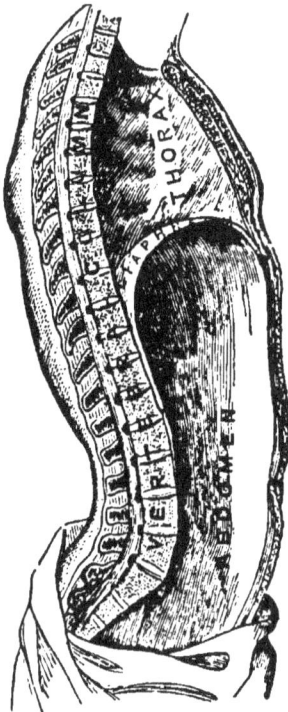

Below the diaphragm — that
is, down-stairs, or in the abdomen
— are the stomach, the liver, the
pancreas, the spleen, the intestines, and the kidneys. These
last-named organs lie behind the
intestines, and you cannot see
them in the picture (Fig. 2).

You can see neither the
whole of the stomach nor its
exact shape. The same is true
of the liver and spleen and the
pancreas ; for these are behind
the stomach, next to the backbone. But you can see the
position in which most of them
lie beside each other, and you
should study the two pictures
(Figs. 1 and 2) till you can
remember their arrangement very well.

FIG. 1. — Side View, showing the
Diaphragm separating the
Chest and Abdomen.

7. **Why the Care of our Health is a Duty.** — We
ought to keep ourselves in good health as far as we
are able, that we may do well the duties of life, and
be useful to others instead of being a burden to

them. Few people can be happy or very useful if they are not well. Every one has some work to do in the world : no one is made to be idle. Some have to work with their hands, others with their heads ; but

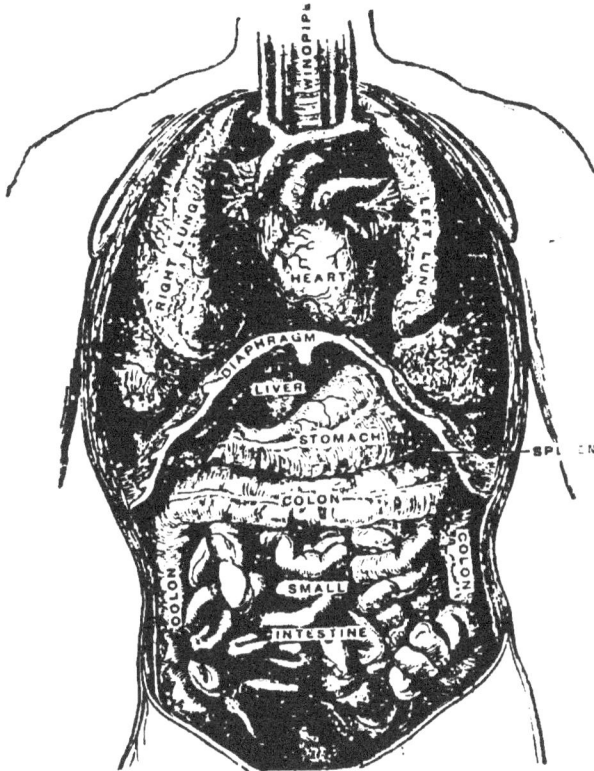

FIG. 2. — Contents of the Chest and Abdomen.

no kind of work can be done well unless the body and the mind are healthy.

To keep ourselves alive, we must have two things, — food and air. But to keep ourselves healthy, the food must be of the right sort, and the air must be pure ; we must be cleanly and temperate ; we must have plenty of exercise in the daytime, and plenty of sleep at night.

If we know the use of the different parts of our bodies, as the lungs, the heart, and the stomach, we shall understand better how to keep them in good order ; just as a man can take better care of his watch if he learns the use of the different wheels and springs.

We cannot be ill without giving trouble to those with whom we live, and causing them expense and loss of time. We cannot prevent all sickness and disease, but a great deal may be prevented when people learn to take care of their health.

Even children may learn many things about the wonderful structure of their bodies. When they grow older they can learn more ; and the more they learn the more they will see that it is a duty they owe both to themselves and to others to do all in their power to keep well.

CHAPTER II

THE BONY FRAMEWORK

8. The Framework of the Body. — The bones are the framework of the body.

They are to the body what whalebones are to an umbrella, what timbers are to a house, or ribs to a vessel. They are the framework of the engine, while the chest and abdomen are the boiler and tender ; our food being the coal.

The brain is like the engineer, who directs all. When he moves a lever, the steam rushes into the machinery, and puts it in motion. When we wish to move, a message goes from the brain to the muscles along the nerves, and the muscles move the bones.

But bones are something more than a framework. They serve many useful purposes. They protect the soft parts which lie beneath them. Thus the bones of the skull shut up the soft and delicate brain in a box of bone, and the ribs protect the heart and lungs in a barrel-shaped cage of bone. Little cups and tunnels are hewn out of hard bone to shield vital organs. Grooves and canals are made in solid bone to shelter tiny blood-vessels and delicate nerves. Even the outside of bones is fitted with little knobs, grooves, and sharp edges, to which muscles and cords are fastened.

In short, the bones are, as it were, a foundation upon which our bodies are securely built.

How many bones do you think we have? Let me tell you. There are in all about two hundred separate bones of various sizes and shapes. Taken together they make the skeleton. We are all familiar with the picture of the human skeleton.

9. **How Bone is made up.** — Bones are very hard and strong. On examining a ham or mutton bone, we would hardly believe there is any soft matter in it. In reality, every bone is made up both of a soft, jelly-like substance, called gelatine or animal matter, and a hard substance, earthy matter, made largely of the mineral known as lime.

Let us show this by two simple experiments. Soak a chicken's leg-bone for three days in a mixture of two ounces of muriatic acid and one pint of water. On taking it out, while the shape of the bone is the same, we find we can easily bend it, like a piece of rubber, or even tie it into a knot. What has taken place? Why, the acid has eaten out the bits of lime, and left only the soft gelatine.

Again : put a soup-bone on the hot coals, and let it burn for three hours. Take it out carefully, and examine it. What do you see? The shape of the bone is the same ; but it is brittle, and will easily crumble between the fingers. Why so? The heat has burned out the soft gelatine, and left only the bone-earth.

In childhood the bones have more animal matter than earthy salts, while in old age they have more lime than gelatine. Hence the bones of children often bend rather than break in the many severe falls they meet with ; while the bones of old people, being brittle, often snap like a pipe-stem with very slight injuries.

The bones are elastic. Thus the Arab children, it is said, make excellent bows with the ribs of camels. The power of bone to resist decay is remarkable. The gelatine — enough to make good glue — will last in a bone for hundreds of years.

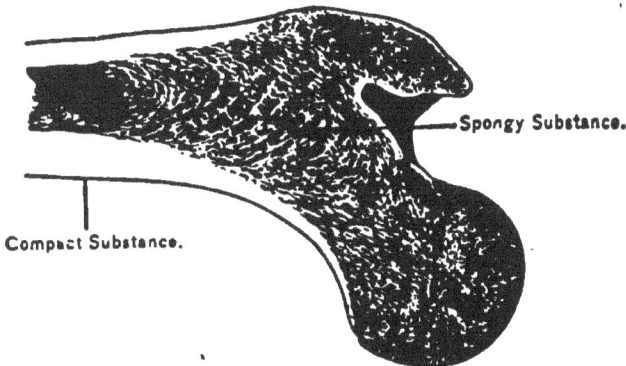

Spongy Substance.

Compact Substance.

Fig. 3. — End of a Bone sawed open, showing the Spongy and Compact Portions.

10. General Structure of Bones. — If we take a long bone, like that from a sheep's leg, or even one end of a soup-bone, and saw it lengthwise, we see that the ends are soft and spongy, while the rest is as hard as a rock. The bone is hollow inside, and filled with a soft, oily substance, called marrow. It is this which makes the flavor and richness of soup.

Crush one end of a bone, and hold it over a hot fire. The heat will soon melt the marrow, which will sputter and burn like tallow. The marrow is the life of the bone. When people speak of a person wanting in energy, they say, " He has no marrow in his bones." The Bible tells us that the " bones are moistened with marrow."

Achilles was a famous Greek warrior of olden times. His teacher, a fabled giant, it is said, fed his pupil upon the marrow of the lion to make him brave. The bones of some animals, like lobsters, are, as you know, on the outside. All our bones are, of course, inside, and are covered with muscles and fat; and over all is the skin.

Again : while we do not cast off our skeleton for a new one every year, as the lobster does, yet our bones are all the time being changed. They are never the same throughout any single hour of our lives. The bones are supplied with millions of the tiniest holes, through which hair-like blood-vessels wind their way, bringing food for the bone, and carrying away waste matters. Thus the blood, " the river of life," oozes its way through every bit of bone as freely as through any other living tissue.

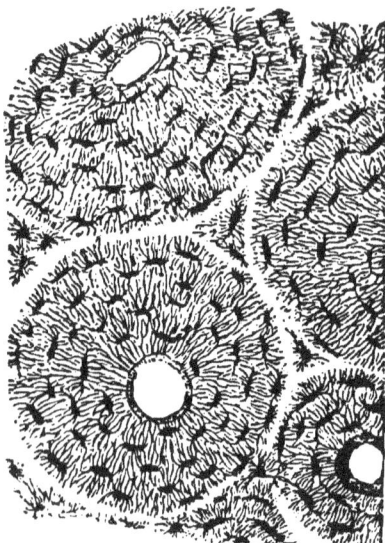

FIG. 4. — Section of Bone as it looks under the Microscope, showing Openings of Canals.

Bones are of many different shapes, according to the uses to which they are put. Some are long and hollow, as the bones of the arm and leg; while others are short, as the bones of the fingers and toes. Some are flat, to cover exposed places, like the knee-pan and shoulder-blades ; while others are of various odd shapes, as the bones of the ankle and wrist, and the backbone.

11. **The Head.** — The **skeleton,** or bony framework of the house we live in, — a house far more wonderful than any king's palace, since it can walk, and the walls are living,— consists of the bones of the **head,** the **trunk,** and the **limbs.** The bones of the head make a very strong box of bone, commonly called the skull. When we speak of the head we mean the head and face.

The top part of the head, which is sometimes called the brain-case, is a kind of bony shell which holds the brain. It is made up of several bones tightly locked together by seams something like the dovetailing

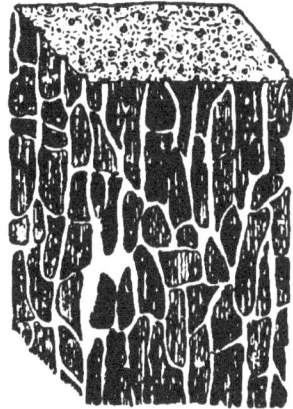

FIG. 5. — Cross Section of Bone, highly magnified ; the Canals are left white.

used by a carpenter. Put your hand on the head of a babe just above the forehead, and you will find a soft space, called a " little fountain." Why is this ?

Simply because, in very young children, these bones, which grow on their edges, do not yet meet, and the throbbing of the brain is easily seen and felt through the thin scalp. Now, as the bones of a child's head are thus dovetailed into each other, they yield a little, and do not break even if he tumbles and bumps his head every day.

All the bones of the head, except the lower jaw, — the only movable bone of the head, — are firmly locked together by these dovetailed stitches, or sutures as they are called. The dome shape of the skull makes it stronger. If you have ever tried the strength of an egg-shell, you can understand what hard blows the head will bear.

Let us see what this box of bone, the cupola of our

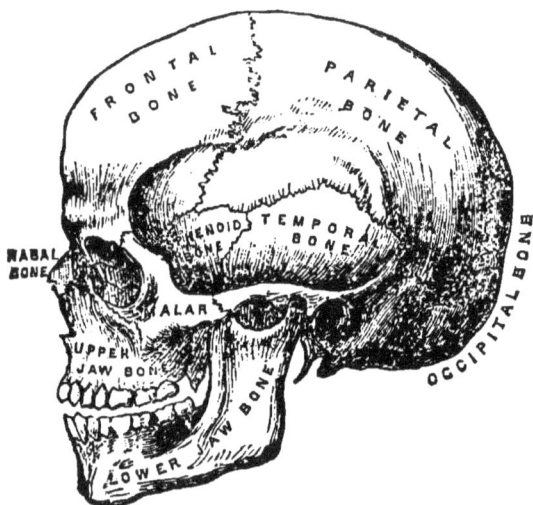

FIG. 6. — The Skull.

bodily house, holds : our eyes, with which we see; our ears, with which we hear ; our mouths, into which we put our food ; the nose, with which we smell ; and then our brain. Indeed, it is a very precious box, we think.

12. **The Trunk.** — The **trunk** is the central part of the body. Let us describe its bones, as those of the **backbone,** the **ribs,** and the **hips.**

The **backbone,** or spine, the main pillar of the building,

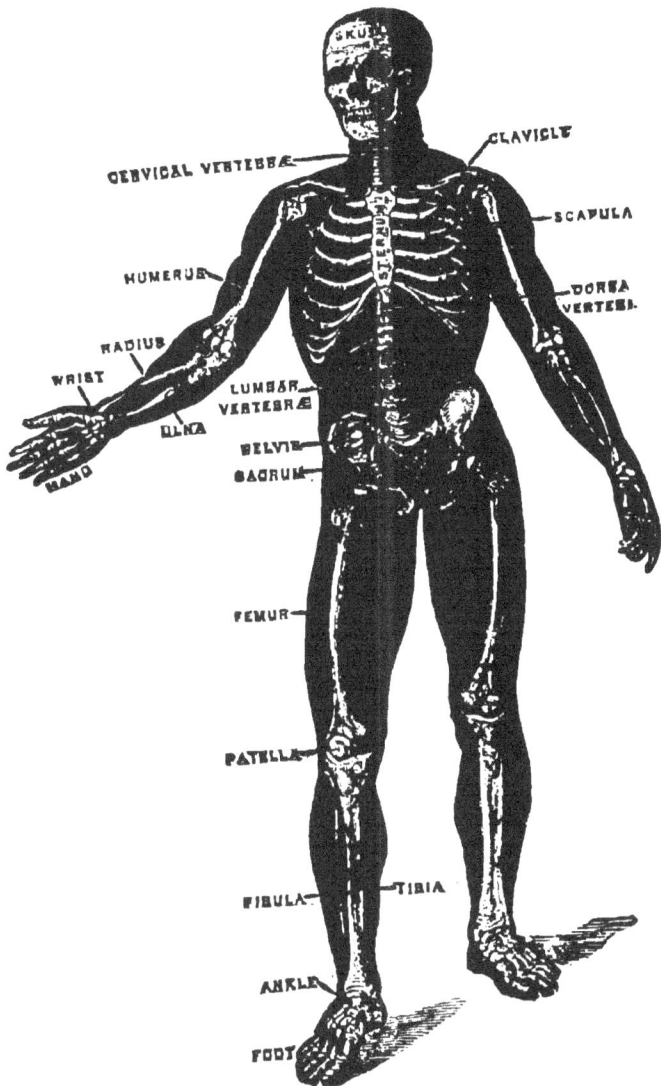

FIG. 7. — Skeleton of Man.

is a tapering pile of separate bones put one on top of the other. The bottom of each fits exactly into the top of the next. Between the bones are little cushions of gristle. They help break the force of any shock or injury to the spine, just as the springs of a carriage lessen the jolting. They also save any wear or tear of one bone on another, and yet allow of their moving pretty freely.

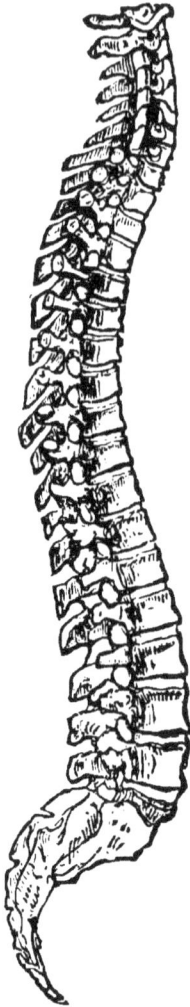

You would hardly believe it, but people who stand or walk much are really a little shorter at night than they were in the morning. A day's work presses together these magic springs ; while a night's rest allows them to expand, so that by the next morning we are as tall as ever. The story is told of a young man who, being just the exact height for military service, walked all night before going up for examination. He gained his point, for he was no longer tall enough to serve as a soldier.

Each bone of the spine has a large hole through it. Imagine a number of spools piled end on end, with the holes exactly over each other. Then there would be, of course, one long hole

FIG. 8.—The Backbone.

through the whole string of spools. This is somewhat the way the bones of the spine are arranged. From each bone of the spine project thorns of bone, to which are fastened muscles which keep the back erect, and lift the head and shoulders.

We can feel these bony ridges by running the fingers up and down the middle of the back. The next time you see a fish on the dinner-table, ask to be shown the large middle bone. It is the fish's backbone; and it will give you an idea of your own, for it is built on the same plan.

The spine is really one of the most curious things in

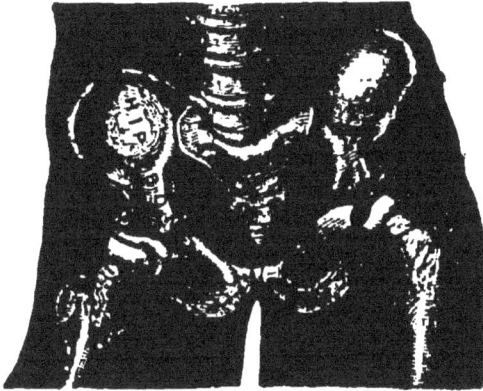

FIG. 9. — The Pelvis.

nature, so firm and yet so elastic, giving the body its graceful form. Think of the great weight which a man can carry on his head with ease and safety. Circus-performers will bend their heads back until they almost touch their feet, thus bringing this curious pile of bones nearly into the shape of a bow.

The **ribs,** twelve on each side, spring from the back-bone, and pass round the chest somewhat like the hoops of a barrel, and are united in front to the breast-bone.

The upper ribs are fixed; the lower ones bend and move when we breathe. If we press our hands on our sides, and take a deep breath, we can feel how much the ribs move.

Every child knows how to rest his hands on the **hips,** the two large, strong bones which make up the lower part of the trunk, — the sills of the house, as it were. Each of these bones has a deep, cup-shaped cavity on its side, about as large as a toy china teacup, into which the round head of the thigh-bone fits.

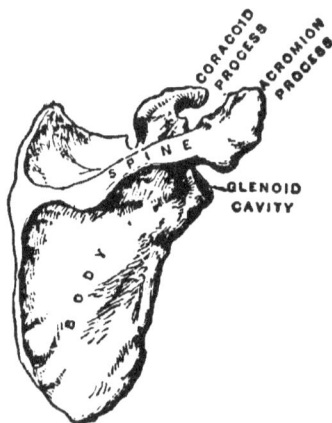

13. **The Shoulder and Arm.** — The shoulder consists of the **collar-bone** and the **shoulder-blade,** the braces of the upper part of the body, one before and one behind.

We can easily feel the collar-bone running across the top of the chest, like a slender cross-beam, over and above the first rib. It is fastened at one end to the shoulder-blade and at the other to the breast-bone.

FIG. 10. — Back of Right Shoulder-Blade.

The shoulder-blade is easily found. Put your hand to your shoulder where officers wear their epaulets, and move your arm up and down. You will feel a bone which seems to dance with every movement of the arm. This is the shoulder-blade. It has a cup-like cavity, into which the round head of the arm-bone fits, and in which it moves with the greatest ease.

The main bone of the **arm** extends to the elbow, where it meets the two bones of the **fore-arm.** Now comes the **wrist,** made up of eight little bones wedged together like the stones of a pavement, only not quite so firmly. From the wrist come the bones of the **hand,** ending with the thumb and fingers. The hand enables us to take hold of anything, as a cane, or to strike a blow when the fist is doubled up. The

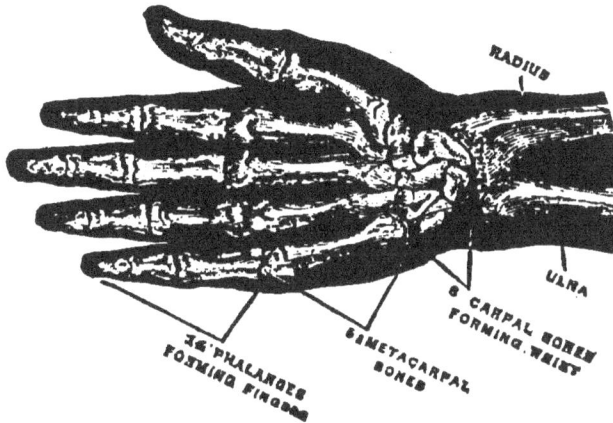

FIG. 11. — Bones of Right Hand.

bones of the hand, wrist, and fingers are held in place by strong but flexible bands and cords. This gives, as you may imagine, a great variety to their motions ; so that the hand can do almost anything that we wish it to do, from grasping heavy hammers, to holding a pen, and threading the finest needle.

It is very curious, that, although the hand of the monkey and the orang-outang seems very much like yours and mine, yet his thumb is on a line with his fingers, and bends in the same direction they do ; while our thumbs are opposite our fingers, giving us a wonderful advantage in grasping and holding objects. Man is the only animal that has his thumb opposed to his fingers.

How wonderful it is that the deaf and dumb talk with their hands, and the blind read with their fingers! Even the most common things that we do with our hands every day are really wonderful. In brief, the arm and hand, with their fifty different muscles and thirty bones, supplied with cords, nerves, blood-vessels, covered with skin, and furnished with nails, make a wonderful set of machinery.

14. The Legs. — How useful are the legs to every other part of the body! Without bones in our legs we could not stand or walk. They are made so strong that they can support the weight of the body, and so light that they are capable of a great variety of movement.

The upper bone of the leg, the **thigh-bone,** the longest and strongest bone in the body, reaches down to the knee. It is so large and so heavy that, in handling it, one might imagine it to be a club; in fact, the warriors of savage tribes sometimes wear the thigh-bones of slain enemies, as a weapon, at their waists.

At the knee-joint the thigh-bone meets the bones of the lower leg, to which it is united by stout cords and bands. A flat, three-sided bone, called the **knee-pan,** fits over the knee-joint in front. You know, if we fall in running, we are apt to strike on the knee. This little heart-shaped bone keeps the joint from getting hurt.

There are two bones in the leg below the knee, — the **shin-bone** and the **splint-bone,** connected with the foot at the ankle-joint.

The ankle contains seven queer-shaped bones, some-thing like those of the wrist, but rather larger.   They are bound firmly together, and are strong enough to bear the weight of the body.

The foot forms an arch known as the instep, not unlike the arch of a bridge, with the heel at the back

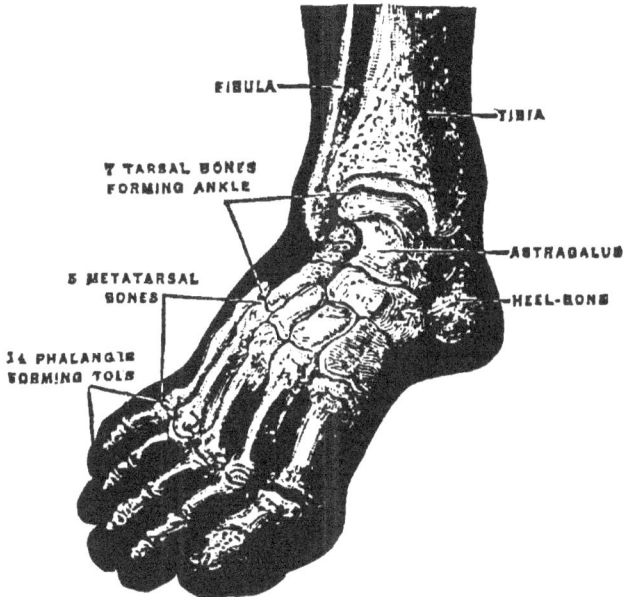

FIBULA

TIBIA

7 TARSAL BONES
FORMING ANKLE

ASTRAGALUS

5 METATARSAL
BONES

HEEL-BONE

14 PHALANGES
FORMING TOES

FIG. 12. — Bones of Foot and Ankle.

and the toes in front.   On this arch the body rests. It is not only very strong, but, owing to the toes being formed by several bones, the whole foot is elastic, and forms a spring by which the body is thrown forward without the other bones being shaken or jarred against each other.

In animals which leap after their prey with a jump or

spring, this elastic character is increased ; and they are
provided with pads under each joint, which serve to
break the shock they would otherwise receive. You
know how quietly and nimbly a cat runs. Now, if you
look at her paws when she has "gloves on," you will
see that this is owing to the little black cushions under
them.

We have, as every one knows, ten toes, — five on
each foot. The toes help us spring in walking. Gristly
bands and cords bind the twenty-six little bones of the
foot firmly together, and yet allow of many different
motions. It is wonderful what habit and necessity will
make the foot do. We who cramp our feet in tight
boots can hardly believe it when we hear of persons
carving, writing, and even painting, with the toes.

A few years ago a French artist used to paint with
his toes pictures worthy of a place in the French Exhi-
bition. Some savage tribes in Australia, it is said, walk
into shallow streams, and catch fish with their toes.
Travellers tell us that certain African tribes steal with
their toes as easily as with their fingers. Chinese
mechanics will pick up tools with their toes, and work
with them while using other tools with their hands.
The Arabs use their fingers and toes at the same time
in braiding ropes.

15. **How Bones are joined together.** — The place
where one or more bones meet and move upon each
other is called a **joint.**

Get a knuckle of ham or mutton at the market, open
the joint by cutting into it, and study what you see.
Our own joints are made exactly after the same general

plan. The ends of the bones, shaped, as you will see, according to the needs of each joint, are moist, and tipped with a smooth, glistening layer of gristle. The next time you have a piece of roast veal on the table examine it carefully, and you will see at the end a white substance, which crackles under your teeth : this is gristle.

Joints are bathed with a sticky fluid something like the white of an egg : the common name for it is joint oil. It allows the rubbing surfaces to move smoothly one on another, thus saving much wear and tear. Think of a man who could build a machine which would last "three-score years and ten" or more, and keep its own joints oiled all the time !

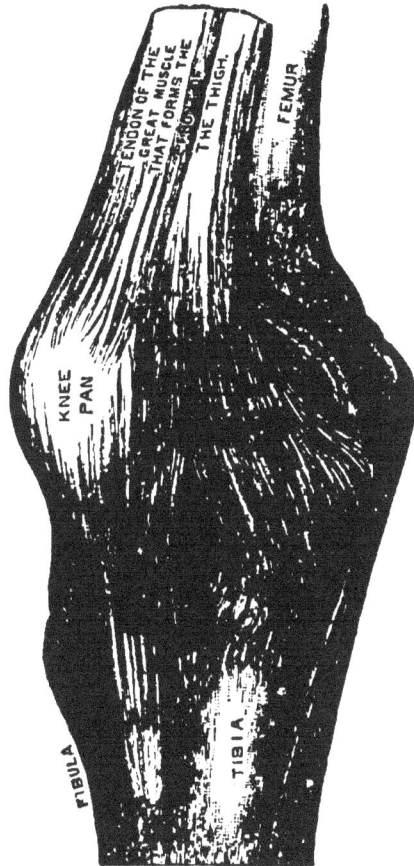

FIG. 13. — The Right Knee-Joint, showing how firmly it is bound about by ligaments.

Some of our joints are real hinges. At the elbow there is a hinge-joint. All the time a carpenter hammers, he uses the hinge-joint at his elbow. All our fingers and toes have hinge-joints. The most curious

joints are called ball-and-socket joints. The head of
the arm-bone, as you know, fits into a cup in the
shoulder-blade. When we move our arms round and
round at the shoulders, we use this joint. A boy uses
this joint all the time he turns a grindstone, or swings
a bat in playing base-ball.

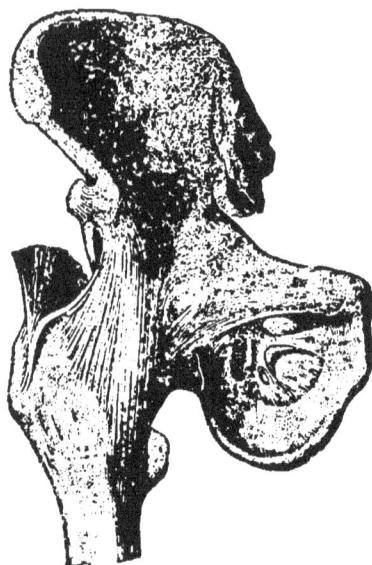

The round head of the thigh-bone, as you already
know, fits into the cup-like
socket of the hip-bone,
thus giving the legs great
freedom of motion. All
these joints are liable to
be put out of their place.
This often happens to the
shoulder-joint, and occa-
sionally to the hip-joint.
Those who play ball, often
put their finger-joints out
of place. We should be
careful not to play at too
violent and rough games,
by which we may not only
put the joints out of place,
but may also break the bones and sprain the cords.
Many children have the habit of pulling the finger-
joints, to make them "crack." This is a foolish custom : it disfigures the hand by enlarging the knuckles,
and, besides, may cause permanent injury.

FIG. 14. -- The Right Hip-Joint.

16. How Bones are tied to Each Other. — If we
pick up two bones that have lain for years, perhaps,
bleaching in the sun and rain, we find that the ends

are smooth, and may fit exactly into each other. · Put the ends together, and they will not stay a moment unless tied together by strings or something of the

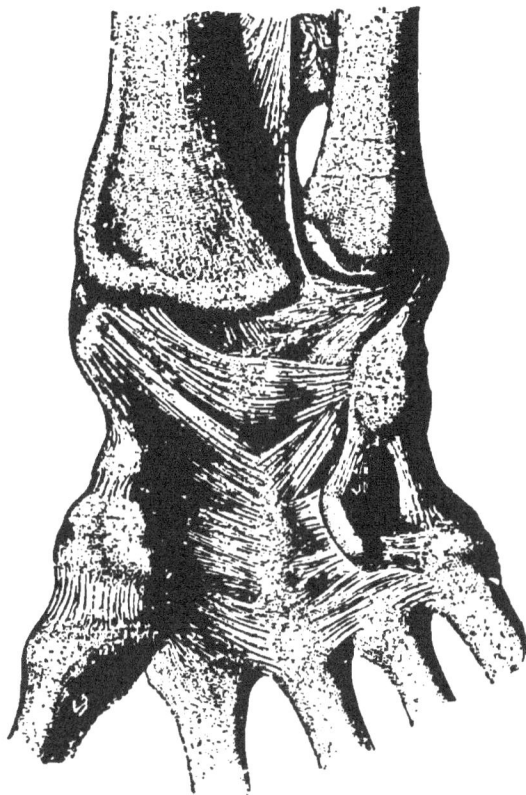

Fig. 15. — Showing how the Wrist- Bones are tied together.

kind. How, then, are the joints held in their places? How are bones kept together in the living person? Simply by strong straps.

Some of them are as narrow as a piece of tape ; others, as at the side of the knee or at the shoulder, are quite wide. Some cross each other, as at the knee-joint; while others shut in a joint, like a bag or sack, thus saving it from being easily slipped out of place. You will find out some day that it takes some skill to carve a turkey or a fowl, because we have to cut round these cords to disjoint it neatly, and serve it out in pieces for the plate.

17. **The Health of the Bones.** — The bones of an infant will easily bend, and even grow out of place, because they are soft and gristly. Stories are told of Indian tribes, the Flatheads, who used to tie small pieces of board, with bands and bandages, firmly on the soft and tender heads of their babies, to flatten them, thinking that a flattened skull of this shape is beautiful. Bones, especially in children, are readily changed by long-continued pressure or strain. You may have heard of the distorted feet of Chinese women. These people think it is low-bred for women to be useful, and have natural feet ; so they bind the baby's feet, if it is a girl, with strong bands, to prevent them growing. When these poor children become women, they are scarcely able to move about.

Did you ever think how hurtful and silly is the fashion of wearing tight and high-heeled boots and shoes ? Why so ? Because high heels throw the weight of the body forward, and force the foot down on the toes. This tends not only to crowd the toes out of shape, causing tender feet, corns, bunions, in-growing nails, and swollen joints, but makes the natural gait stiff and ungainly.

Knowing the practical importance of having comfortable feet, Frederick the Great kept a servant whose foot was exactly his size, and made him wear his new shoes till he himself could wear them with comfort ; and, poor fellow, he sometimes wore them too long, and got kicked by his royal master for his pains. The Duke of Wellington, being asked once as to the most essential article of a soldier's clothing, replied, "A good pair of shoes."— "What next ?"— " A spare pair of shoes." And even thirdly, "A spare pair of soles."

Children should not be allowed to walk too early, before their legs are strong enough to bear the weight of the body. The soft bones may bend, and cause "bow-legs," so commonly seen on the street. Children should not get into the habit of taking hurtful positions, such as sliding down into the seat, or sitting on the foot. Bending over too much while reading, writing, sewing, or otherwise at work, is apt to cause round shoulders.

At school the desks should not be too low, thus causing a forward stoop ; or too high, thereby throwing one shoulder up too much, and giving a twist to the spine. If the seats are too high, the feet have no support, and injury to the thigh may result ; if too low, there is undue strain on the shoulder and backbone. Round shoulders and curvature of the spine may result from long-continued positions of this kind. Seats should be regulated according to the size of the pupil, and frequent changes should be made.

18. Effect of Alcohol and Tobacco on the Bones. — As the bones grow they need material for building them up. This material has to be carried to them by the blood. If the blood is made poor or poisoned with alcohol or tobacco, the bones are deprived of the matter they need for their growth. Physicians are agreed that tobacco tends greatly to stunt the growth of the bones.

Many boys are dwarfing their bodies as well as their minds, by smoking cigarettes. No boy can afford to lose a part of his growth, for the sake of a habit that does him no good, and that makes him an object of disgust to cleanly people.

CHAPTER III

THE MUSCLES

19. **Our Muscles.** — We move and walk from place to place by means of our muscles. Our limbs are moved by the muscles. Muscles move not only the limbs, but the skin. Watch the horse, and see him shake his hide to get rid of the biting flies. Our bones, our fingers, and toes, our mouth, our eyelids, — all are moved by muscles. In short, all motion in our bodies is dependent upon them.

Muscle is simply lean meat or flesh. When we eat beefsteak or lean mutton for dinner, we are eating muscle.

FIG. 16. — A Muscular Bundle teased out to show its fibres.

When corned beef is boiled very tender, so it falls apart, we can easily divide it into strings: these strings are muscular fibres. See how they are glued together, into bundles of various shapes, by a very thin web not unlike the thinnest of thin tissue-paper. Each bundle is called a muscle. We may compare a muscle to a handful of tiny skeins of silk packed into bundles, and dividing again and again until they are

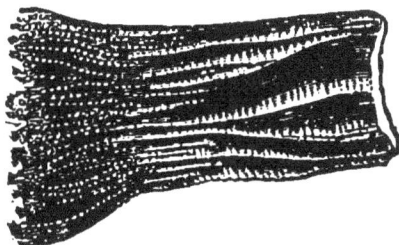

a thousand times finer than the finest hair on our
heads.

Muscles are of all sizes and shapes. Some are
large, others very small; some are shaped like fans,
others like quill pens; many are broad and flat in the
middle, and taper down at each end. In brief, the
shape of muscles varies according to the place where
they are put and the work they have to do.

Sometimes we can see the shape of the muscles
through the skin, especially in
the arm and shoulder of a man
who does hard work. See the
brawny arm of the blacksmith
as he works at his forge. Look
at those large muscles, strong
as iron bands, that swell out as
he brings his hammer down on
his anvil.

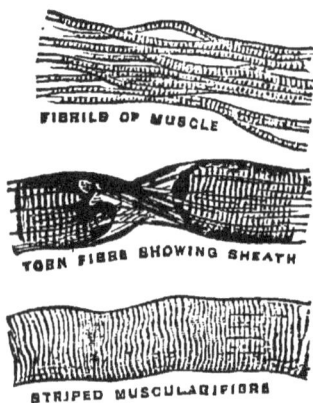

20. **How the Muscles do
their Work.** — Muscles have a
peculiar power of their own
which no other kind of tissue
in the body has. This is the power to become shorter
and thicker. We see something like muscular action
in a piece of india-rubber. If we take a piece of
this, and pull it out longer, we see that it becomes
thinner; and when we let it go, it snaps back, and once
more becomes short and thick. This is very much like
the action of our muscles; but muscular tissues do
this by their own peculiar power, without being pulled
by some one else, as a piece of india-rubber must be.

FIBRILS OF MUSCLE

TORN FIBRE SHOWING SHEATH

STRIPED MUSCULAR FIBRE

FIG. 17. — Portions of Muscular Fibre
highly magnified.

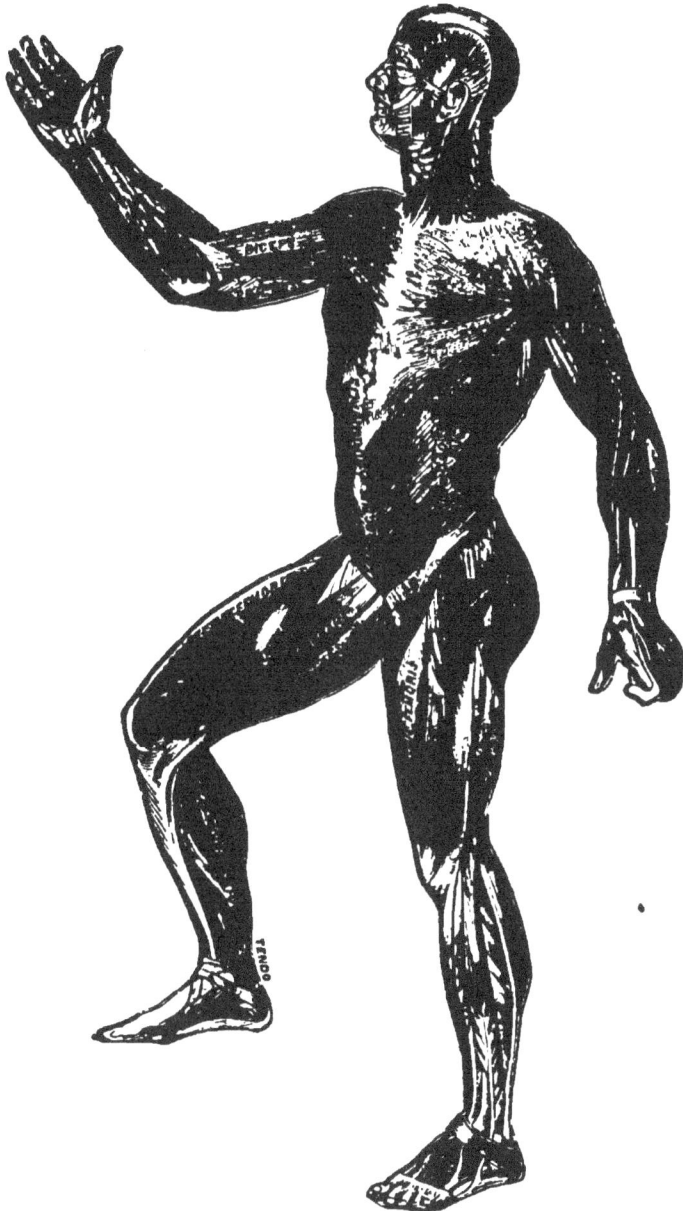

FIG. 18. — Showing Principal Muscles of the Front of the Body.

Now, let us see how this power in our muscles enables us to move. Let us notice what happens when we bend the arm, as boys do "to try their muscle." You will understand that all similar actions — such as clos- ing the hand, opening the mouth, lifting the leg, and so on — are done practically in the same way. Stretch out your right arm, and grasp it above the elbow with your left hand, half way to the shoulder. Now bend your right arm briskly up and down, and feel the big

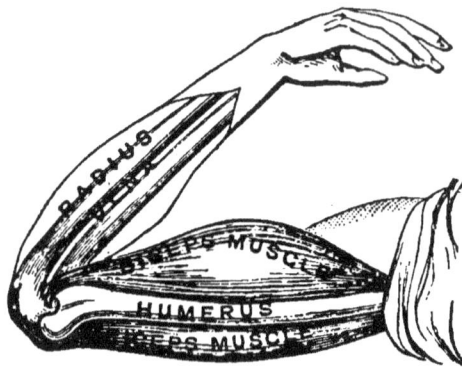

FIG. 19. — This figure shows the Biceps Muscle contracting so as to draw up the arm. When the arm is again straightened the Triceps has a swollen appearance, because it has contracted and become thicker.

muscle on the front of the arm swell and harden as you hold your hand upon it. What has happened? Let me tell you.

When we wish to draw up our hand toward our shoulder, the brain sends a message to the muscle; and the muscle at once becomes thicker and shorter, and pulls up the fore-arm towards the shoulder. Watch the bare arm of a strong man while he pulls up his hand to his shoulder, and you will see the muscle swell up as it becomes thicker and shorter. In this way almost all our movements are made.

This is muscular action ; and this growing thicker and shorter, by which the action is done, is called the contraction of a muscle.

All muscles act in this way by contraction, though, of course, all the muscles are not fastened to bones. Thus the tube by which food passes from the mouth to our stomach is made of rings of muscle. These rings contract, one after another, and so the food is pushed by a worm-like motion into the stomach. So one of the muscles of the mouth is in the shape of a ring. This enables us to pucker our lips.

21. Some Muscles not under the Control of our Will. — There are some muscles in our bodies, however, not under the control of our will. We do not mean to say that they are not controlled by the nervous system, but simply that they are not directed by our brain at first hand. In brief, these muscles do not need to have a message come from the brain telling them what to do.

Let us study this a little. The stomach, for instance, which digests our food, is made of this muscular tissue which our will does not control. As soon as we swallow a mouthful of food, and it passes into the stomach, the nerves feel that it is there, and cause the muscles to begin to act in the proper manner for digesting it. Thus food is digested whether we are willing or not.

The heart, which pumps the blood, is another of these muscles which serve to show us the reason why they act without our will having to order them. We know that the heart is always beating. If we lay our hand on our left side, there it is, *thud, thud,* never stopping so long as we live. If it stops, we shall die. Now, if we had to will every beat of our heart, how dreadful it would be! We should not be able to think about anything else. Years ago a man lived in Ireland who could, by an effort of his will, cause his heart to stop beating for a few moments. He at last lost his life in the act.

Remember, then, that many important organs, made of muscular tissue, but intended always to do some special work, are under the management of nerves, but not of that part of the brain through which our will acts : while other muscles which have to do different things at different times, such as those of our hands, our feet, our eyes, and our lips, are under the control of our will, and do what we bid them.

22. The Tendons. — Some of the muscles are fastened directly to the bones, and grow, as it were, into them. As a general thing, however, muscles are not themselves fastened to bones, but taper into white, tough cords, called **tendons.**

Put your hand in the hollow of the knee, and you will feel something like cords which you would almost mistake for bones when they stiffen. If we put our fingers on the front part of our wrist, and then work our hands and fingers, we feel some cords just beneath the skin. These are tendons, the little ropes with which the muscles in the fore-arm pull the hand and fingers.

Again : if we bend our fingers to and fro, we can see the tendons move on the back of the hand. Children at Thanksgiving time often amuse themselves by pulling the white cord in the leg of the turkey, and seeing

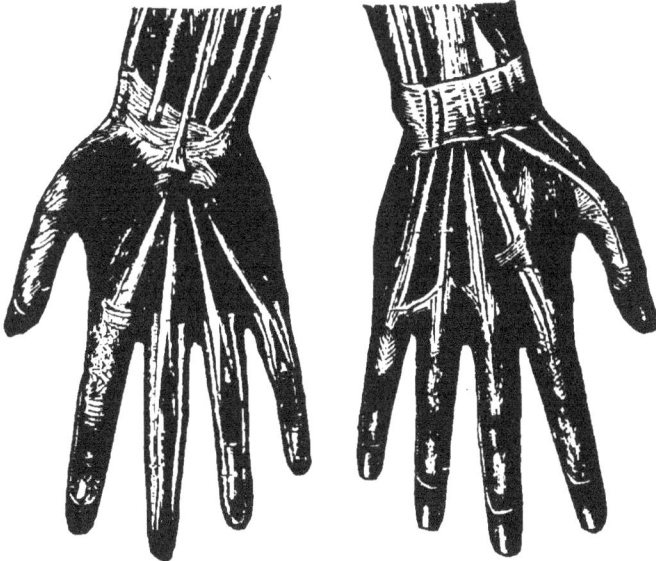

FIG. 20. — Showing the Muscles and Tendons of the Hand.

its toes move. Tendons are most numerous about the joints, especially the larger ones, like the knee and elbow. They save a great deal of space, and allow great freedom of movement where muscles large enough to do the work would be bulky and clumsy. What a large and clumsy foot we should have if all the muscles which are needed to pull the toes were in the foot !

The longest and strongest tendon in the body is just back of the ankle. It is called the tendon of Achilles, after the Greek hero of that name. According to one story, Achilles received his death-wound in the heel, no other part of his body being liable to injury.

23. Why we need Exercise. — Every part of our bodies ought to be used if we wish to be vigorous and healthy. You know what stout, strong arms a blacksmith has: that is because he uses them so much. Constant use, instead of wearing them out, as it would if they were tools, does them good.

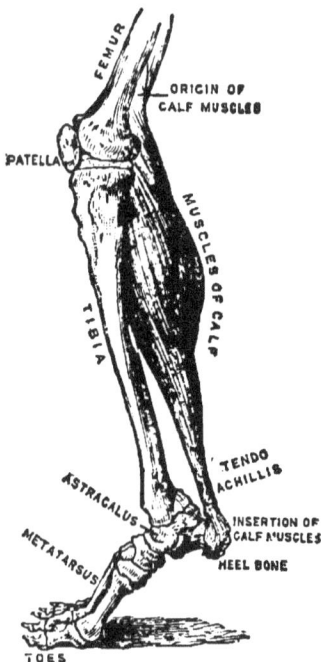

It is just the same with other parts. A person who uses his eyes as he ought has good eyesight, and sees many things another person cannot see. A person who uses his ears as he ought comes in time to hear many things another person does not hear. We are told that savages, who are always looking and listening with all their might, either for enemies or game, have parts of their eyes actually larger than ours, just as a blacksmith's arms grow larger by constant use.

Any part of our body that we do not use finally becomes weak and helpless. Let the blacksmith

FIG. 21. — Bones of Leg and Foot and Muscles of Calf.

change his work for that of a clerk, and the once brawny arms become smaller and weaker. We read of certain people in India who, as an act of worship, keep one arm raised above the head until the muscles shrivel and become useless.

All the parts of the body have so much to do with each other that each one has some effect on all the others. Now, what we commonly call taking exercise — that is, walking, running, and jumping — not only strengthens our arms and legs and backs, but makes our blood flow faster and brisker. It makes us breathe in a great deal more fresh air, it helps us to get rid of more waste matter, it makes us warm and comfortable, and it keeps our digestive organs in good order.

In brief, **exercise** makes us stronger and better all over.

What a good thing it is for boys and girls that they are so fond of play! Playing base-ball, running races, skipping with a rope, — all these games help them to grow up into active, healthy men and women. The old adage says, "Change of work is as good as play." There is a sense in which it is quite true. If we have been sitting and reading a long time, it rests us to get up and take a walk. If we have taken a long walk, it rests us to sit down and read. In these ways change of work is as good as play, because it is a real change, and exercises quite a different part of our bodies.

24. **Time for Exercise.** — The best time to take exercise is about two hours after a meal. It is not best to do hard work or take severe exercise before break-fast. Those who go to work, or study, before breakfast,

should first eat a little plain food, or even drink a glass of milk, just enough to "stay the stomach." Just after a full meal the stomach is busily doing its duty :

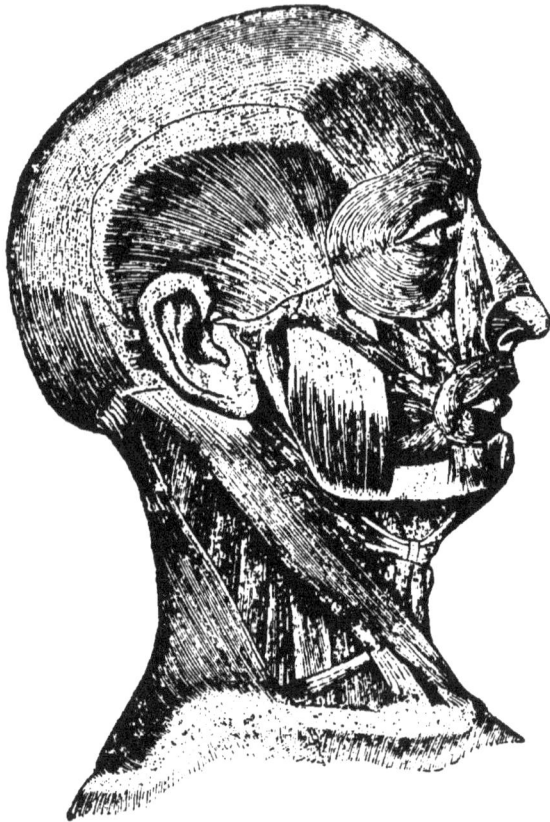

FIG. 22. — Muscles of the Face and Neck.

hence severe exercise at this time is apt to hinder its action, and results sooner or later in ill digestion.

The evening is not the best time for exercise, because the body is tired after the labor of the day. It is useless to make any exact rule for any one person. Ordinary work or moderate exercise, as walking, is healthful at almost any time, except just after a full meal.

25. Different Kinds of Exercise. — The kind of exercise depends very much upon one's daily work. Persons who sit at desks, stand at counters, or work in close rooms, as clerks, teachers, tailors, and printers, are apt to suffer from a lack of bodily exercise and from foul air. Every person should learn by careful observation to know his own needs and his own dangers. All sound persons should every day do some work or take some exercise with both body and mind. To get and to keep vigorous health, it is not at all necessary to increase the size of our muscles very much, or to do great feats of strength.

Walking is the best of all exercises. It takes us into the open air and the bright sunlight ; it puts new life into many important muscles of the chest, abdomen, and limbs. With a brisk walk every day, taking care to keep warm and dry, no one need suffer from lack of proper exercise.

Running, leaping, climbing, and other vigorous sports, are well enough if we do not get over-tired. Violent sports, such as base-ball and foot-ball, are severe exercises, and occasionally dangerous.

Rowing is admirably suited to most persons of either sex. Horseback riding, coasting, swimming, and skating are important helps to increase bodily vigor.

The quick and graceful gymnastic exercises practised in many of our schools are especially healthful,

and should be more generally used. Growing children
should be trained every day, at home or in school, in
the use of light wooden dumb-bells, light clubs, or
wands. A daily exercise of ten minutes will do much
to develop feeble and narrow chests, to check a tendency
to curvature of the spine and round shoulders, so common with young people, and to give strength and vigor
to all parts of the body.

One of the simplest and most useful modes of light

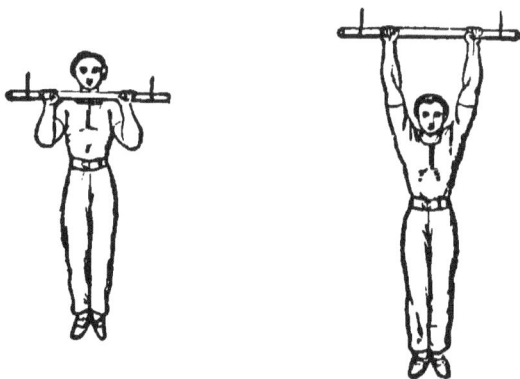

FIG. 23. — Exercise on the Swinging Bar.

gymnastics is to fasten a broomstick in some suitable
place in your house, suspending it securely over your
head as high as you can reach. Exercise several times
every day in this way : swing, hanging by both hands ;
after a while with one hand, and drawing the body up
to the stick.

Rubber straps and rings, sold in the shops for this
purpose at a trifling cost, are convenient helps in light
gymnastic exercises.

26. Effect of Alcohol on the Muscles. — The muscles are connected with the brain by nerves, and through these nerves the brain controls the action of the muscles. Now, as we shall learn hereafter, alcohol deadens the nerves. Therefore when a person drinks more or less alcoholic liquor, the muscles are acted upon in a peculiar way. Why so? Because the nerve-force that governs the muscles is weakened, and they show a lack of control.

The nice movements required in the handling of fine tools for delicate work, or for gymnastic feats, need steady and well-trained muscles that are under perfect control of the brain. Tippling with alcoholic liquors deadens the nerves that connect the brain and muscles, and thus impairs this control, and, therefore, injures a man's ability to do fine work. This injury results in proportion to the amount of alcohol taken. The drinker may know the right way of making each movement, but he cannot make his muscles move as they ought. He is clumsy, and lacks precision.

Thus we see that under the influence of alcohol, the trained muscles become feeble and trembling, and are no longer wholly under the control of the will. The degree of this loss of control varies greatly with the individual, with the kind of liquor, the rate at which it is taken, and many other circumstances.

This same lack of control is shown in the act of speech. After drinking alcohol, there is less control of the muscles of the tongue and throat : hence words are left out, cut short, or misplaced.

If the person continues to drink until he reaches the

point of intoxication, his nerves become more and more
deadened, and he gradually loses more and more of
the control of his muscles, until finally even clumsy
movement is impossible, and he is said to be dead
drunk.[1]

27. Effect of Alcohol on Strength. — A drink of
beer, rum, or any other alcoholic liquor, cannot increase one's strength for extra hard work, as some
people seem to think. Trials made with the "health
lift" and in other ways show that alcoholic drinks
weaken instead of strengthen the muscles.

A number of workmen were once divided into two
companies, each engaged in the same kind of work.
For a week the men in one company took no alcoholic
drinks of any kind : the men in the other drank as
usual. Before the end of the week the men who were
using no alcohol found they could do more work with
less fatigue than when they drank beer. The next
week the other company of men made the same trial,
and with the same result.

The recent war in the Soudan showed that the
British soldiers could endure the hardships of war in
that hot country better without alcohol than with a
regular ration of strong drinks. Experience has
taught the same lesson to the Indian porters of South
America. When they travel upon their hard journeys
with heavy loads upon their backs, they are careful to
take no alcoholic drinks with them.

Men who are in training for boat-racing, base-ball,
foot-racing, and other sports where great exertion is
called for, are not allowed to use alcoholic liquors.[2]

[1] See note 1, page 229.   [2] See note 2, page 229.

28. Effect of Tobacco on the Muscles. — Tobacco causes weakness and unsteadiness of the muscles. Applicants for the position of book-keeper are frequently rejected because of the tobacco habit, which shows itself in their unsteady handwriting. One of the first things demanded of a young man who is going into training for a foot-race is to stop smoking.[1]

[1] See note 3, page 231.

CHAPTER IV

WHAT WE EAT AND DRINK

29. Why we need Food. — Our bodies, as you have been told before, are in some respects like a steam-engine. Our food is to us what coal is to the engine. Like the locomotive, our bodies move about, and are warm, because a fire is always burning in them. This fire, like that of the engine, needs fresh fuel from time to time. Without fuel and air, the fire in the engine will go out.

So it is with our bodies : without food and air, the bodily fire would soon go out, and we should die for want of them. When coal or wood is burned, we get ashes. So, too, in our bodies : we produce not exactly ashes, but something like them, which must be got rid of, else the fire would flag.

Again : each and every part of the steam-engine is always wearing out. So it is with our bodies : we are all the time wearing out. Every beat of the heart, every movement of a muscle, the wink of an eyelid, and the twist of the tongue, even our very thoughts, — all these lead to waste. Every step we take, every word we speak, wastes a little bit of our bodies. In short, we are working and wasting all the time, at the expense of some tiny portion of the body.

Then, why do we not waste away? We weighed this morning just as much as we did three days ago; some of us, we hope, a little more. How can this be? Why, we have been doing something else, part of the day, besides working and wasting. This something was to eat our dinner yesterday and our breakfast to-day. This is the whole story. What we eat and drink takes the place of what is used up or wasted. If we are young and growing, we must take in a little more than the actual waste.

Nearly all this waste is made good by our **food** and **drink;** the rest of it comes from the air we breathe.

The food we eat, you will think, does not look much like our bodies, of which it is to make a part. Perhaps we may think the meat is rather like it ; but how about bread, milk, butter, and potatoes? How are all these things turned into flesh, hair, and bone? How, indeed, does it ever get to them, — to our knees, fingers, toes, and eyes, for instance?

Let me tell you in four words : *the blood carries it.* The blood not only carries away the waste matter *from* every part of the body, but also brings nourishment *to* every part. In brief, as the Bible says, " The blood is the life."

30. Tissue Foods : the Albumens. — What a great variety of articles we eat and drink ! Is this a good or a bad thing? A good thing, as we shall soon see. Many unnatural things are eaten for food in certain parts of the world. Thus certain tribes of Indians in South America eat a peculiar kind of clay.

Beetles were eaten by Roman epicures, and are said

also to be eaten by Turkish women to make themselves fat. Bees, moths, ants, mice, and many small animals, form staple articles of diet in other countries. Humboldt, the great traveller, tells us that centipedes are eaten eagerly by some of the natives of South America. Locusts and grasshoppers are eaten by the Digger Indians in the West.

We can easily put all ordinary foods into three great groups. First, we have certain kinds of food to make up for the wear and tear of the body ; that is, **tissue foods,** or **albumens,** so called because they build up the tissues.

They are called albumens because they contain a whitish substance called albumen. The white of an egg is a familiar illustration : it is almost wholly made up of albumen. Lean meat, the cheesy part or curd of milk, pease, and beans are rich in albumen. Wheat, barley, oats, rice, and corn also contain albumen. All these foods hold something which our muscles and blood especially need, and which we are using up and getting rid of it every moment. Hence, to make good this loss, we must eat tissue-making food, or else we should slowly starve to death.

31. Fuel Food : the Sugars and Starches. — Now, while some foods are chiefly useful as flesh-formers, — that is, they mainly go to make new flesh and new bone, — other foods more especially make heat, and enable us to do work. These fuel or heat-giving foods we may divide into two classes, — the **sugars** and **starches,** and the **fats.**

We might, perhaps, think that all our sugar comes from sugar-cane, and must be bought at the grocer's ;

but this is quite wrong. There is a little sugar in wheat, and a good deal in some other things we eat, such as pease, oatmeal, beets, honey, milk, grapes, watermelons, and many other articles. Sugar is very easily digested; it is dissolved in the mouth by the saliva, and then passes down the food-pipe into the stomach, where it is taken up by the blood-vessels. In the blood parts of the sugar combine with other substances in the body and make heat.

The sugars and starches form a large part of all those plants commonly used as food. Wheat, barley, rye, oats. rice, corn, arrowroot, sago, and potatoes are rich in starch. In its natural state starch is useless as food until it has been acted upon by the digestive fluids.

When starch is well chewed, it is changed into sugar by the action of the saliva. This is why a piece of bread tastes sweeter after it has been in the mouth for a few minutes. Old people with poor teeth, and young people too, indeed, often like the crust of bread, or the heel of a loaf, especially if it is soaked in milk or tea. Why? Because it is sweet; and it is sweet because, having been baked harder, the starch has been partly changed into sugar. We seldom, however, keep the food long enough in the mouth to change all the starch of our food into sugar; this is done farther along in the act of digestion, as we shall soon see.

32. The Fats. — Some people, especially children, do not like fat; some of us may have a feeling of disgust at the mere thought of it. But we all must eat fat in some form or other. We are familiar with this class of food, under the names of pork, fatty meat, suet, lard, butter, olive-oil, and cod-liver oil.

Fat is a heat-giving or fuel food. For this reason, fatty foods are much used by people who live in cold countries. The Esquimaux, who live in Greenland, drink one or two quarts of oil, and eat several pounds of tallow candles, every day. Their children, it is said, have as keen a relish for tallow candles as our children have for bananas or ice-cream. Sir John Franklin once tried to find out how much fat an Esquimau boy could eat. Fourteen pounds of tallow candles quickly disappeared ; and Sir John, feeling alarmed for his stores, closed the experiment with a large piece of fat pork.

Oil is a luxury greedily devoured by the Northern races, as was amusingly proved in a seaport town some years ago. The town was lighted with oil-lamps, and it was noticed that they went out early for several successive nights. At last it was discovered that some Russian sailors in the harbor climbed the lamp-posts and drank the oil.

Once upon a time some English sailors made a "Christmas-tree" for some Esquimau children by tying together some walrus-bones, and hanging on them balls of whale-blubber, instead of bonbons. This was a rare treat for the children, who ate the balls of fat as eagerly as we would eat chocolate-creams.

33. The Mineral Foods : the Salts and Iron. — All the foods we have just studied come from living things, as animals and vegetables. Besides these, we must eat certain things which have no life, and never had. We will call these **mineral foods.** First of all, water is a mineral food; but this will be described more fully hereafter.

We cannot do without common salt as an article of food. All nations, both civilized people and savage tribes, eat it daily, both by itself and along with other food. The lower animals like it too. Farmers put lumps of salt in their fields for the sheep and cows to eat. Wild animals flock in great numbers to places known as salt-licks.

Men have risked their lives to get even a taste of salt. In olden times untold tortures were inflicted upon prisoners by feeding them on bread alone, and that made without salt. In most countries it "is as cheap as dirt," while in parts of Africa it is worth its weight in gold. Salt has always been the symbol of life, hospitality, and wisdom; and the Scriptures tell us, "Salt is good. Have salt in yourselves, and have peace one with another."

How much salt do you suppose we have in our bodies? About half a pound, but we are all the time losing it. Tears, we know, contain salt; and it is also found in the sweat. Some may think they do not eat any salt, because they do not eat it by itself. But we must remember that many foods we eat, as meat, oatmeal, and cheese, have just a little of it.

Now, we need some other salts to help purify the blood. These are the salts of potash, found in the vege-tables, especially lettuce. Sailors who have been forced to go for a long time without fresh vegetables always suffer much from a fearful disease called scurvy. In Lord Anson's celebrated expedition round the world,

which left England in 1740, four out of five of the
original crew died of scurvy. Again, we all need,
especially growing children, salts of lime to make the
bones harder and stronger. This is one reason why
children should eat plenty of bread and milk.

Would you think that we need any iron in our food?
Well, we do; for it is iron that helps to make good
blood, and to color it a bright-red hue. Iron in small
amounts is found in many of the foods we eat.

34. Water as a Food. — Pure water is our great
natural drink. Many savage nations know no other
drink, and require no other. Water helps to change
our food into the blood, dissolving it in the stomach
just as it would in a glass. A lump of sugar put into
a glass of water soon disappears, but we know it is still
in the water by its sweet taste.

Not only is the greater part of our drink water, but
bread, meat, potatoes, fruits, and other foods, also have
water to make them easy to digest. Nearly three-
fourths of the weight of our body is made up of water;
in fact, every tissue and organ in the body is watery.

How important it is, then, to have the water we
drink pure and fresh! We are all the time getting rid
of a great deal of water, — nearly two quarts every day,
—through the skin, lungs, and kidneys; hence we
must take in water every day to make up for this loss,
besides what we drink. Certain foods, as lettuce, cabbage, apples, fish, potatoes, and lean meat, are more
than three-fourths water. Water alone will prolong life
if nothing else can be had.

A few years ago, as some of us remember, it was

claimed that Dr. Tanner lived forty days without taking any other food or drink than water. There is a well-known case of a miner who lived twenty-three days, buried in a coal-mine, without swallowing anything but water sucked through a straw.

35. Important Articles of Diet. — The most important food is bread, "the staff of life," without which we should indeed be poorly off. There is no single food in the world which meets so many real wants of the body. Bread may be made from the flour of many kinds of seeds, — such as wheat, oats, barley, rye, and Indian corn ; but in this country it is nearly always made from wheat.

Wheat-flour gives us starch, sugar, and a kind of albumen called gluten ; hence wheat has nearly everything to support life, except fat. When we eat bread and butter, we have nearly a perfect food.

Corn-meal is a highly nutritious and cheap article of food. Oatmeal and milk is a very cheap and nutritious article of diet. The famous Dr. Johnson once spoke of oats as "food for men in Scotland, and horses in England ;" and a sturdy Scotchman added, "Yes, indeed ; and where will you find such men and such horses ?"

Rice, though rich in fat-making food, is one of the least nutritious of all the cereals. Pease and beans contain more tissue-making food than any of the cereals, and are as rich in starch as is wheat-flour. The common or Irish potato is a most important article of diet ; although it is more than two-thirds water, and has little nutriment, yet it is easily digested, and is a cheap and economical article of diet.

Ripe fruits, such as apples, pears, peaches, melons, grapes, and oranges, though not of much nutritious value, are prized for their agreeable flavor. Sugar and molasses are both largely used in cooking and confectionery.

Among animal foods milk is the simplest and best. It is, indeed, a model food. It has flesh-forming, bone-making, and heat-giving material in the right proportions, especially for children. What a wonderful thing is an egg! It has a great amount of nutriment packed away in the smallest space, and is easily digested. Its value as food is equal to that of the same weight of meat.

Meats, for the most part, consist of the muscles of the various animals. The most common are beef, mutton, lamb, veal, and pork. Meat is rich in albumen, and has more or less of fat. It is a most important article of diet, and, as a whole, is easily digested, except, perhaps, veal and pork. Fish is at once a cheap and nourishing food. Poultry is easy to digest, and gives a deal of nourishment, especially for the sick. Like all fats, butter is almost entirely a heat-giving and force-making food. Cheese is nutritious, but is not easily digested.

36. Artificial Drinks. — Man has always contrived many ways to flavor his drink. The greater portion of almost every drink is water, but in various ways other substances are mingled with it to give it a pleas. taste. Tea, coffee, cocoa, beer, wine, and distille liquors are the more common artificial drinks.

Some persons, however, cannot drink a single cup

coffee or of tea without feeling the worse for it ; headache, indigestion, heartburn, wakefulness at night, are the most common effects.

Strong tea in large quantities should never be used. Hard-working women and others too often make their meals of dry toast and several cups of strong tea. Such a habit is sure to result in indigestion. Taken in large quantities tea may weaken the action of the heart, and produce the peculiar beating, after much exertion, known as palpitation ; hence we have the "tea-drinker's heart." Coffee and tea are hurtful articles of diet for growing boys and girls, and doubtless all would be in better health without them.

How often do we see people, over-heated and over-tired, drink glass after glass of ice-water ! Such a foolish habit often leads to serious results. Ice-water quenches thirst only for a moment. Sooner or later it weakens the strongest stomach. If you must drink it, sip a little very slowly.

As you already know, the most common artificial drinks are alcoholic liquors. In the next -chapter we shall learn a great deal about their origin and nature.

CHAPTER V

ORIGIN AND NATURE OF FERMENTED DRINKS

37. Sweet Apple-Juice. — When the juice of apples is first pressed out it is sweet. A kind of sugar forms in apples while they are ripening. This gives the juice its sweet taste. Very soon after the apple-juice is pressed out, unless it is kept very cold, it begins to change and to lose its sweetness. Why? Because the sugar of the juice is being changed into something else which is not sweet but strong and poisonous.

38. Ferments and what They do. — What causes the apple-juice to change? Let me tell you: it is due to minute forms of plant life called **ferments**. These rest on the skins and stems of the fruit. When the apples are ground up these ferments are washed into the juice. If our eyes were strong enough we might see them on the outside of the apples before they are ground, or floating about in the air ready to fall into the juice as soon as it is pressed out.

A single ferment could not do much harm; but when one gets into fruit juice in a moderately warm air it begins to produce rapidly new ferments like itself. Thus in a few hours after the juice is pressed out it will contain countless numbers of ferments, each rapidly putting out little buds that become new ferments, while they at the same time change the sugar of the juice into two substances entirely different from sugar.

The gas which you can see coming up out of the liquid in little bubbles is one of these substances; the other is **alcohol,** a poison. You do not see the alcohol because it mixes with the apple-juice and remains in it.

39. Alcohol. — Alcohol is a poison[1] which in sufficient quantities will cause death; in small quantities, its poisonous effects may show themselves more slowly, and thus escape notice for a time.

40. Alcohol and Water Contrasted. — Alcohol looks like water, but its nature is very different from that of water. Water will not burn; alcohol will. Water poured on a plant will cause it to grow and thrive; alcohol poured on a plant will kill it. A fish which lives all its life in water would die at once if put into alcohol. Every part of our bodies needs water; we should soon die if we could not get it. No part of the body needs alcohol; thousands of people die every year from taking it into their bodies.

Water softens our food and helps it to digest; alcohol hardens many kinds of food. Water soothes and refreshes the body, outside and inside; alcohol inflames and irritates every part of it. Water quenches thirst; alcohol creates thirst. It is the nature of alcohol to create in one who takes it a desire for more. This is as true of small quantities as of large.

41. The Appetite for Alcohol. — Alcohol has the power to create an appetite which will lead a man to sacrifice health, property, ability to work, the respect of his friends, and everything that makes life worth living,

[1] See note 4, page 232.

for the sake of obtaining drinks that contain the deadly poison. This is called the **alcoholic appetite.** This appetite is not like the ordinary appetite for food. It is a diseased craving, the result of injuries that the alcohol itself has caused.

The appetite for food is a natural appetite. When enough food is taken to supply the wants of the body for the time, the appetite is satisfied. The same is true of thirst. When enough water is drank to supply the need of the body in health, no more is wanted. But every drink taken to satisfy the craving for alcohol leaves behind a worse craving for more.

Men who have devoted years to trying to rescue those who have become victims of the appetite for alcohol say that, with all their efforts, only a few are finally saved. Men who have abstained for months or even years may be suddenly overpowered by the slightest taste or even smell of an alcoholic drink.

Drunkenness is due more to the nature of the drink than to the weakness of the drinker. The greatest weakness of the drinker is in beginning to take the drink that has the power to make him its slave.

42. Alcohol as a Flavoring for Food. — It is the custom of some housekeepers to use wine or brandy as a flavoring for jellies, pudding-sauces, mince pies, and other delicacies. Knowing what we do of the nature of alcohol, it is easy for us to see how wrong and danger-ous is such a practice. It may create a taste for alcoholic drinks, or arouse an inherited or acquired taste in one who is trying to overcome it.

43. The Law of Fermentation. — The process by which the sugar of a sweet fruit or plant is changed to alcohol is called vinous **fermentation.** There are other kinds of fermentation, produced by other kinds of ferments. Each fermentation has its special kind of ferment, but one law holds good for every kind. It is this : —

FERMENTATION ENTIRELY CHANGES THE NATURE OF THE SUBSTANCE FERMENTED.

Thus if cider is left standing in a warm place, another kind of ferment gets into it, and changes the alcohol into a new substance, entirely different from alcohol or sugar. This new substance is acetic acid, and the liquid containing it, which was first sweet apple-juice, and then cider, is now vinegar. There is no alcohol in vinegar.

44. The Evils of Cider-drinking. — The fermented drink made from the juice of apples is called **cider.** When the juice is first pressed out, it is said to be "sweet cider." As it grows older, more and more alcohol forms in it, and it is then said to be growing "hard." Hard cider is often one-tenth alcohol.

A mistaken idea very commonly held is that cider only a few days old contains such a very small quantity of alcohol as to be practically harmless. Experience proves that even such cider has enough alcohol in it to arouse the thirst for stronger drinks in one who is trying to break off from their use. In moderately warm weather, alcohol is found in cider in about six hours after it has been pressed out. We need not go far to find those who have been led to drunkenness by cider, for a little alcohol in cider or in any other drink has the power to create an appetite for more.

Cider seems also to have the power to make the drinker ill-tempered. It is a marked trait of cider-drinkers that they are cross and ugly in their dispositions.

45. Wine a Dangerous Drink. — Ferments are found upon the skins and stems of grapes as they ripen. If the juice of the grapes is then pressed out, the ferments are washed into it, and turn the sugar of the juice into gas and alcohol. The gas will escape in bubbles while the alcohol will remain in the liquid. Such a liquid is called **wine.** We do not see the alcohol in the wine ; but it is there, and can be separated from it as we shall soon learn. We can also trace its presence by its effects upon those who drink the wine.

We must remember that wherever alcohol is found its nature is the same, and that it gives its harmful qualities to any liquid containing it.

It is an error to suppose that because grapes are good, a drink made by fermenting their juice is also good. We have learned that fermentation changes the nature of the substance fermented. Vinous fermentation changes healthful grape-juice into poisonous wine by changing its sugar, which is a food, into alcohol, which is a poison.

The alcohol in wine is capable of creating an appetite for more alcohol. In Persia, France, Switzerland, California, and other countries where wine is made, drunkenness is a great scourge, especially during the wine-making season. It has been claimed that the use of "light wines," i.e., wines containing only a small amount of alcohol, prevents drunkenness ; but in countries where such "light wines" are as free as water, the drunkenness resulting from their use shows that there is no foundation for such a claim.

The tendency of drinking wine, or any other liquor containing alcohol, is to lead to drunkenness.

46. Beer and its Dangers. — Fermented drinks containing alcohol are made from liquids having in them a certain kind of sugar like that in fruit juices. This kind of sugar can be obtained from starch by keeping it warm and moist for a certain time. Barley and other grains containing starch are therefore used to make one kind of fermented liquors called "malt liquors." In making these barley, or whatever grain is used, is kept warm and moist until it begins to sprout, which is the sign that its starch has turned to sugar.

It is then heated to kill the sprouts, ground, and soaked in water; and in this way a sweet liquid is obtained. Yeast, which is one kind of ferment, is then put in, and hops which give the liquid a bitter taste. The yeast changes the sugar of this grain-juice to alcohol and a gas. The gas bubbles up to the top where it leaves a froth. The alcohol remains in the liquid, which is now called **beer.**

Beer is used as a drink by many people who do not understand its real nature, or who have only learned its nature after having formed such a liking for it that they cannot easily give it up. It has been called "liquid food" because it was thought that the substances which make the grain good for food were in the beer. But, as we have seen, fermentation changes the nature of the sugar obtained from the starch of the grain.

In this change nearly all the food value of the grain is destroyed and a poison is left in its place. The man who eats the bread he could buy for the price of a glass of beer, and drinks pure water, gets real nourishment and no poison.

47. Beer no Preventive of Drunkenness. — It has been urged that a more general use of beer would prevent the drunkenness caused by drinking the liquors that contain more alcohol, such as rum, whiskey, brandy, and gin. We have only to look to the countries where beer is used in nearly every family, to see that it is no preventive of drunkenness. True to its nature, the alcohol in the beer makes the drinker crave more beer to get more alcohol. In Germany, Belgium, and other countries where beer is almost a universal beverage, drunkenness is becoming more and more a curse to the land. What is lacking in quantity of alcohol in the beer is made up by the quantity of beer drank.[1]

48. Beer gives a False Appearance of Health. — A stout, healthy-looking brewer's drayman boasted that he had drunk a gallon of beer every day for the last thirty years, and that he was never in better health than at that moment. The next day he died of apoplexy. It is a fact well known to physicians and surgeons that a small cut, which on a healthy person would heal in a short time, on the beer-drinker, who may look the very picture of health, often becomes a dangerous wound from which blood poisoning and death may result. A prominent London physician says, " A copious beer-drinker wears his heart on his sleeve, bare

[1] See note 5, page 233.

to a death wound even from a rusty nail or the claw of a cat."[1]

49. Beer-drinking from a Moral Point of View. — Facts gained from wide observation show that beer more than any other liquor tends to make the drinker brutal. It seems to deaden conscience and blunt the finer sensibilities, and thus prepare a man for committing crime.

The fact that beer contains less alcohol than some other drinks is no argument in its favor when we remember that the nature of alcohol is the same wherever or in whatever quantity it is found. The alcohol in even the weakest beer has the same power of creating an appetite for more that an equal quantity of alcohol in any other liquor has.

50. Fermentation in Bread-making. — Fermentation is employed in making bread. The flour from which the bread is made contains a small quantity of free sugar. Yeast is mixed with the flour and water, and the dough is kept warm and moist until the yeast changes this free sugar to alcohol and gas.

But the fermentation is soon stopped, and the alcohol is driven out by the heat of the oven in which the bread is baked, while the gas, pushing its way up through the dough, makes the bread light. To get this light sponginess is the purpose for which the yeast is used.

Thus we see that no one need to be afraid to eat bread raised with yeast, through fear of its containing alcohol; for well-baked bread contains no alcohol. You may be sure that bread never gave any one an alcoholic appetite.

[1] See note 6, page 234.

51. Distilled Liquors. — When water is heated to a certain temperature it begins to turn into steam. Alcohol will turn to vapor at a lower temperature than water. Therefore, by heating a fermented liquid the alcohol in it can be readily driven off in the form of vapor. This is condensed in a cool receiver, and the result is a liquid containing much more alcohol than the one heated. Some water will follow the alcohol, for alcohol has a special liking for water. This process is called **distillation.**

Brandy is distilled in this way from wine. Rum is distilled from the fermented juice of the sugar-cane ; whiskey from a fermented liquid made from corn and rye ; gin from rye or barley. Distilled liquors all contain a large proportion of alcohol, often as much as one-half. They lead to the swift destruction of whoever drinks them.

CHAPTER VI

DIGESTION, AND HOW IT GOES ON

52. What is meant by Digestion. — When a sick
person is very feeble indeed, especially from the loss
of blood, the doctors sometimes do a remarkable
surgical operation : they open the sick person's vein,
and inject warm milk or beef-tea, or perhaps fresh
blood directly from another person's veins. They
inject enough of this to revive the sick man, and
thus perhaps save his life. But no one would ever
think of feeding a person many days in this unnatural
way. Of course, the best way to be fed is by the good
old mode of eating and drinking.

A part of what we eat is not nutritious, and would
clog up the body instead of feeding it. The waste
part of the food, therefore, must be got rid of ; but
the nourishing part, after it has gone through many
changes, and has had some things added to it, becomes at last the living fluid called blood. Can anything be more wonderful than that flesh and vegetables, and bread and water, and other things that have
no life in themselves, should, when once taken into
the body, change into living flesh, living bone, living
skin ?

The process by which food is thus made fit to mix with the blood is called **digestion.**

In a general way, we may compare this process to a vegetable-garden, where side by side, from the same soil, grow pease, corn, tomatoes, pungent horse-radish, and sharp peppers, — and poisonous weeds by the fence on the edge of the garden.

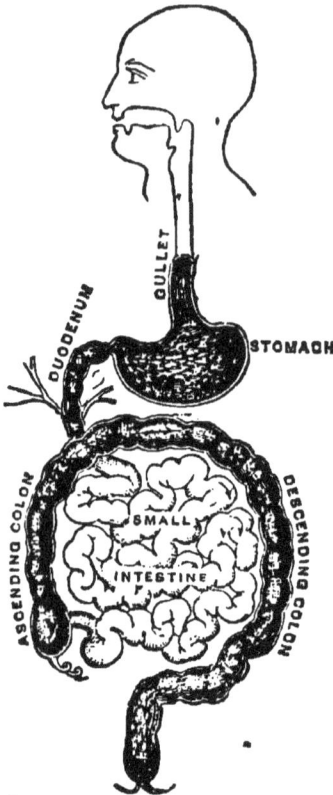

53. What takes Place in the Mouth. The Teeth.—The food is broken into pieces in the mouth by the teeth, — valuable little jewels, of which the jaws are the jewel-cases. During our lifetime we have two sets of teeth. The first set, twenty in number, begins to appear when a child is about six months old. A child may really be born with teeth. Some day you will read in your history that Louis XIV., a great king of France, Richard III., a wicked king of England, and Mirabeau, a famous French orator, were born into the world with teeth.

Fig. 24. — Diagram of the Digestive Canal.

When we are about six years old, the first set, commonly called the milk-teeth, drops out ; and the second or permanent set of teeth, thirty-two in number, gradually takes its place. Each tooth is set down into a socket in the jaw-bone, like a post in a hole. The teeth are coated with a thin layer of a very hard substance, called enamel. Each tooth has inside a fine tube filled with blood-vessels and nerves. When a tooth is decayed, and the nerve is open to the air, it makes it ache. As some of you know, it hurts to have a tooth pulled out.

54. **Mixing the Food with Saliva.** — The food, chewed by the teeth, is rolled around by the tongue,

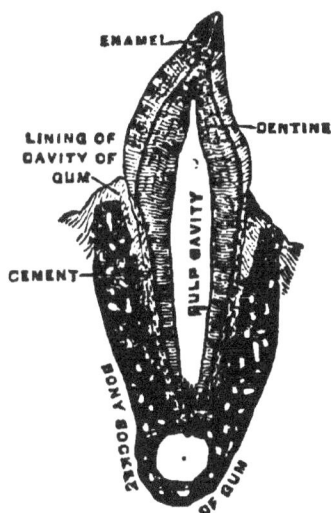

The teeth of one-half the jaw separated.

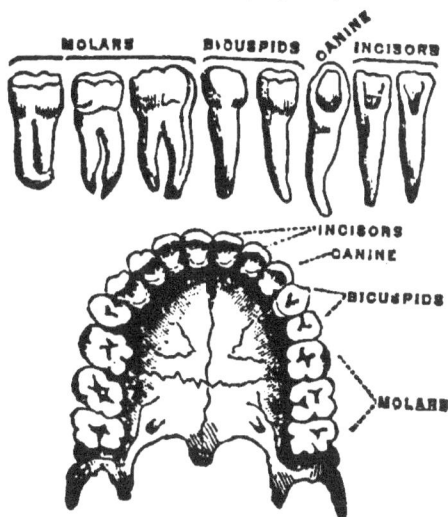

ENAMEL
LINING OF CAVITY OF GUM
DENTINE
CEMENT
PULP CAVITY
BONY SOCKET
OF GUM

MOLARS   BICUSPIDS   CANINE   INCISORS

INCISORS
CANINE
BICUSPIDS
MOLARS

FIG. 25. — Vertical Section through a Tooth lodged in its Socket.

FIG. 26. — The Teeth.

hard pressed against the roof of the mouth, and then swallowed. During this time the food is well mixed with the fluid of the mouth, called **saliva,** which flows from a number of little spongy organs inside the mouth. Probably you have had the "mumps," or at least have seen some friend who has had the disease. What is it? Why, sometimes these little organs, of which there is one under each ear, become inflamed, and grow large ; and this is known as the "mumps."

The saliva wets the food, and so makes it easier to swallow. It has, besides, another very important work to do : it acts on the starchy part of the food, changing some of it into sugar. You know that a piece of bread grows sweet in the mouth when it is well wet

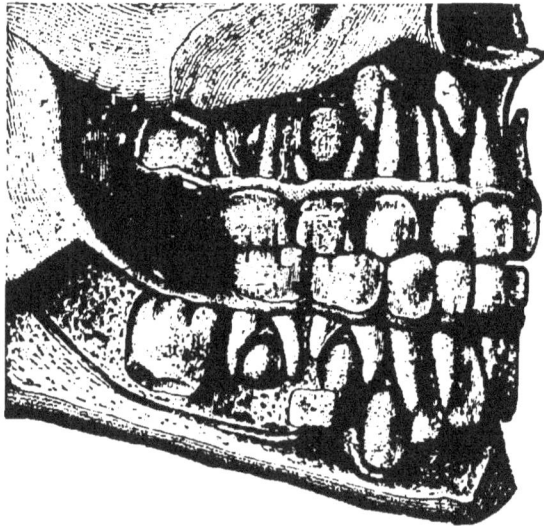

FIG. 27. — Section of Jaws, showing the Milk and Second Teeth.

with saliva. This work of the saliva is important, else starch could not be dissolved, and therefore would do us no good as food, while sugar is readily dissolved.

When we are not eating, the saliva flows only in small quantities, just enough to keep the mouth comfortably moist ; but when we begin to eat, these little factories do a brisk business, and pour into the mouth a large quantity, about half a pint, it is said, at a single meal. The sight, or even the thought, of a savory dish, will make the saliva flow, or, as we say, "make the mouth water." The sight of a piece of meat will make the saliva run out of a hungry dog's mouth. Run your finger to and fro in the mouth several times, and notice how quickly the saliva flows.

Smoking and chewing tobacco cause an undue amount of saliva to flow from these glands, thus making the mouth dry. The constant spitting of tobacco-juice wastes the saliva needed to digest the food, and after a time causes ill digestion. Fear will stop the flow of saliva : hence in India they try sometimes to detect a thief by making those who are suspected chew rice. The person from whose mouth it comes out dryest is judged to be the thief.

We can now understand how necessary it is to chew our food well with our teeth before swallowing it. If we eat very fast, and bolt our food nearly whole, we get little good from it. It does not digest easily, and sooner or later we shall suffer for our negligence.

55. How the Food is swallowed. — The food is now ready to be swallowed. The soft, moist mass, pushed into the back of the mouth, is forced down the **gullet,** or food-pipe, by a peculiar motion something like the waving of the skin of a worm's body when it is crawling. If you watch a horse's neck when he is drinking, you will see the peculiar motion along his food-pipe. A wave of motion follows just behind the food and pushes it down.

Another hollow tube, in front of the gullet, opens into the back of the mouth, — for you know it is as necessary to breathe air into our lungs as it is to take food into our stomach, — and this other tube, or wind-pipe as it is called, is therefore for the air to go down. If the food were to slip down the wind-pipe instead of the food-pipe, we should be choked to death. We all know, when a bit of food goes "the wrong way," how we have to cough until we get it up. In order, then, to prevent mistakes, the top of the wind-pipe is protected by a trap-door.

A very clever fellow this little trap-door is. When we are just going to swallow a morsel of food, down it goes quick and tight, and keeps the food out of the wind-pipe; but, as soon as the food is down, up jumps the trap-door, so as to let air pass down to the lungs. This wonderfully useful little servant does not have any common name, but is called the *epiglottis*, meaning "upon the tongue."

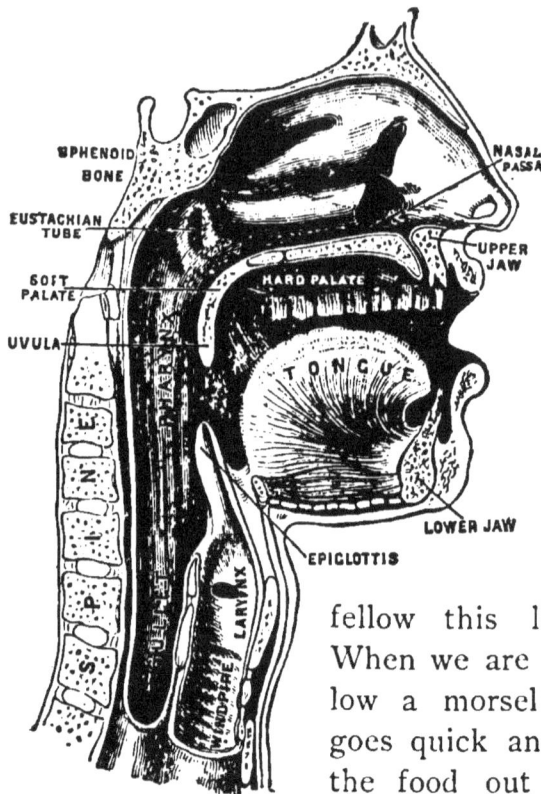

FIG. 28.—Section showing Passages to the Gullet and Windpipe.

56. What takes Place in the Stomach. — The food, a moistened, partly digested mass, has now reached the

stomach.   The **stomach** is a pear-shaped bag, capable of
holding about two quarts.   It lies across the upper part
of the abdomen, a little toward the left side.   The size
of the stomach depends upon what there is in it.   As
we fill it with food, it swells out larger, like a toy balloon, which becomes smaller or larger according to the
amount of air in it.

The stomach has two openings, — the gullet end,
through which the food enters, and the out-going end,
a kind of muscular
ring.   This out-going
end, called the " gate-
keeper," is made in
such a wonderful
manner that any food
trying to get through
too soon is sent back
again, so that only
properly digested
food is allowed to

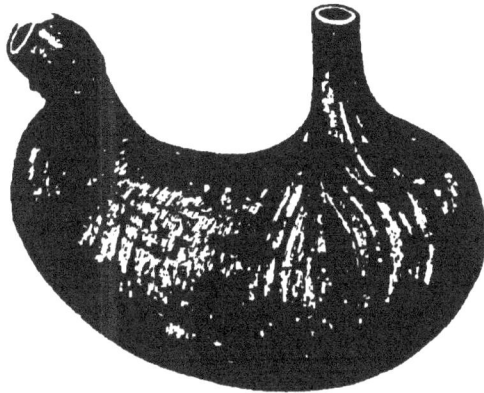

FIG. 29. — The Stomach.

pass.   Would not that carpenter be called a very clever
man who could make a door which would open and shut
of itself at the right time, which would let only the
right sort of people go in, and would crowd away the
wrong ones ?

As we begin to eat, the walls of the stomach stretch
themselves out to make room for the food, and begin to
move gently with a wavy motion, which carries the food
round and round, as if it were being churned.   This
churning motion is slow and gentle at first, but gets
faster and faster as digestion goes on.

As soon as the food arrives in the stomach, thousands of tiny glands in its walls pour out on the food a fluid called the **gastric juice.** This flows in great abundance — several quarts, probably, every day, — and has in it a peculiar substance, called "pepsin," which is necessary to the digestion of food in the stomach. The gastric juice dissolves, and thus helps digest, that part of food which has albumen in it, — the lean meat, gluten of flour, and so on. A part of the contents of the stomach, being easily dissolved, and so already sufficiently digested *in* the stomach, need not go any farther, but passes at once into the blood. The way in which it gets from the stomach into the blood is very curious indeed. All over the walls of the stomach on the inside are thousands of very small blood-vessels with very thin walls. The dissolved food soaks out of the stomach through these very thin walls into the blood-vessels and so reaches the blood. The food not dissolved in the stomach, and needing further digestion, passes into the intestines.

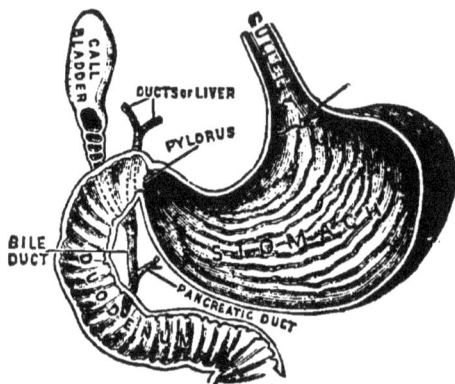

FIG. 30. — Section of Stomach.

If we could only see all these wonderful things going on inside of us, especially in the stomach ! It would be more instructive than watching the bees make honey through the glass windows of their hives. Well, do

you know that the inside working of a man's stomach
has really been watched through an opening in his side?
About sixty years ago a Canadian named Alexis St.
Martin was accidentally shot in the left side. After
much pain and suffering he recovered; but the opening
into the body never quite healed up, but remained a
kind of window through which his doctor could look in
and see what was going on in his stomach. The doctor
saw the gastric juice
pour in upon the
food, and he found
that some things
were much more
easily digested than
others. He also dis-
covered that, when
the young man ate
things which were
unwholesome, the in-
side of the stomach
became red and in-

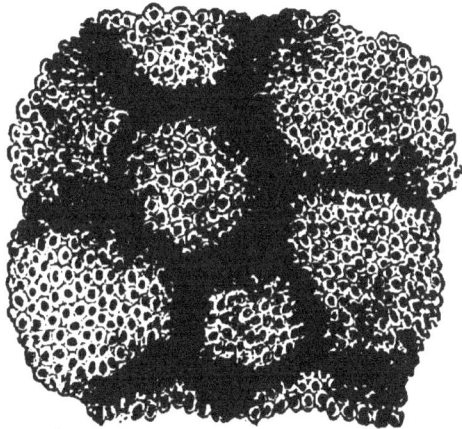

Fig. 31. — The Inside of the Stomach, showing the
Opening of the Glands, highly magnified.

flamed, and did not do its work properly. Thus we see
that the stomach has a great deal of hard work to do;
it is a busy workshop, where all that is eaten is partly
made ready for the use of the body. It was a favorite
saying of Frederick the Great, that "an army moved
on its stomach."

57. How the Intestines do their Work. — When
the food has been properly prepared in the stomach,
the gate-keeper of the stomach opens the gate for the
partly digested food to pass out into the long tube

known as the **intestines,** or the bowels. This tube is about thirty feet long, but it is so rolled up and folded away in the body that it takes up very little room. In the first foot of the intestine, the food is mixed with two fluids which flow into it through two little pipes.

One is of a greenish-yellow color, called the bile, which is made in the **liver.**

The other, called pancreatic juice, by the **pancreas,** or sweetbread, as we call it in animals.

The liver is so important a part of our bodies, that we must learn a few things about it. It is the largest organ in the body, and weighs about five pounds. It is on the right side, in the upper part of the abdomen, and its lower edge is sometimes easily felt just below the ribs.

The **bile** is made by the liver, and stored up in a little pear-shaped bag attached to the liver, called the gall-bladder. This little bag is made aware, in the twinkling of an eye, when the food enters the first part of the intestines, and straightway pours out its greenish fluid. The next time the cook cleans a fowl, ask her to show you the little greenish bladder which she calls the gall, and which she takes care not to burst, because it holds a bitter fluid which, if spilt upon the fowl, would quite ruin its flavor.

The liver is a very busy workshop; in fact, it does double duty. It is the great rag-picker of the body. It makes, out of the waste matter of the blood, the bile which is so necessary to our health. Again, the liver is a storehouse, storing up a kind of sugar, which is gradually doled out to the blood as it is needed for the use of the body.

The fat we eat is not digested in the mouth or stomach, but in the first part of the intestine. The bile helps divide the fat into the tiniest pieces, and so fits it to be taken up by the blood. The fluid from the sweetbread also aids in the digestion of fat, finishes the digestion of the starchy foods not already changed into sugar by the saliva, and carries on the digestion of other foods which the stomach has failed to do.

58. How the Blood feeds on the Food. — Now that the food has been acted upon by the digestive fluids, and has become a thick, creamy mass, it remains for us to see how the rich, nutritious part is to get into the blood.

This is done chiefly by two sets of vessels, — the **blood-vessels** and the **lacteals** or **lymphatics.**

The process by which the digested matters are taken into the blood is called **absorption.**

The inner lining of the digestive tube is richly supplied with blood-vessels. Certain parts of the food can readily soak through the delicate walls of these vessels, and so are taken directly into the blood.

The inside lining of the intestines is not smooth, like the outside, but has a velvety appearance. Millions of short, velvety threads, called "villi," meaning tufts of hair, hang down, like very small tongues, into the inside of the intestines. They are tiny affairs, about one-thirtieth of an inch long, and a five-cent piece would cover five hundred of them. They have the look of the pile on plush. We are, of course, familiar with this appearance in tripe.

In each one of these villi is a network of the finest blood-vessels, and a tube called a lacteal, meaning "milky," because it carries a white, milky fluid. Millions of these lacteals dip down into the intestines.

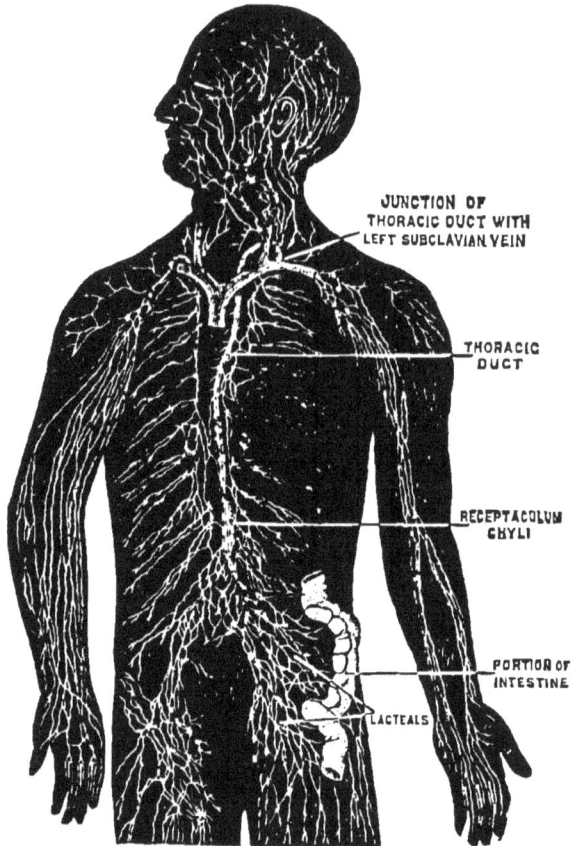

FIG. 32. — Lacteals ending in Thoracic Duct, which empties into a Vein in the Neck.

like little root-fibres, and suck up, like so many open mouths, the fatty matters of the food from its creamy contents. The lacteals, after passing through a num-

ber of glands in the abdomen, like way-stations on a
railroad, unite into larger tubes, and finally open into
a little sac in the loins.

Leading upward from this is a tube about eighteen
inches long and about as large as a lead-pencil, called
the **thoracic duct**, which carries the fluid upwards beside
the backbone, and pours it into a large vein situated
close to the heart.

Now we must remember that absorption has really
to do with a work of far wider character than that of
merely keeping the lacteals busy. The lacteals are
simply those lymphatics which have their roots in the
villi of the intestines. In all parts of the body, except
the brain, spinal cord, eyeball, and tendons, we find
thin-walled vessels busily at work taking up, and making over anew, waste fluids or surplus materials derived
from the blood and tissues generally. They seem to
start out of the part in which they are found, like the
rootlets of a plant in the soil. The tiny roots join
together, and make larger roots. They carry a colorless fluid called **lymph**, very much like blood without
the red corpuscles.

The tubes in which this fluid flows are called
lymphatics. These tubes have rounded bodies at many
points of their course, scattered along like depots along
a line of railroad, called **lymphatic glands.**

They seem to be factories to make over the lymph in
some way, and fit it for renewing the blood. Most of
the lymphatics at last unite with the lacteals, and
empty their contents into the thoracic duct. Thus,
Nature, like a careful housekeeper, uses up even the

waste matters of our bodies, in providing them with nourishment.

The nutritive matter thus absorbed from the food leaps into the blood-current, carrying with it a renewal of life and power. The life of the body is thus, as you see, supported by the nutritive part of the food, every drop of which will turn into blood, — the blood which flows through our hearts, nourishes our limbs, and is flushed into every nook of our bodies.

The lower part of the intestines is a kind of temporary storehouse for undigested and waste matter, which must be got rid of as speedily as possible.

59. How much to eat. — The quantity of food needed to keep the body in good health varies very much. The greater the amount of exercise, the more food is needed to make up for the waste. During the time of growth, a still greater quantity is needed to build up new tissues: hence growing children generally have a good appetite and a vigorous digestion. The same holds good of persons getting well of some long and wasting sickness.

The quantity required also depends very much upon one's business. Those who work hard and long, either with the body or mind, as teamsters, blacksmiths, farmers, doctors, and editors, need a goodly amount of nutritious food. Those who work in-doors, as clerks, milliners, students, and bookkeepers, can get along with a smaller quantity. In cold weather and in cold climates, a greater quantity of fuel-food is necessary than in warm weather and in a tropical climate.

An appetite for plain, well-cooked food is a safe

guide to follow. Every person in good health and
with moderate exercise should eat well ; he should

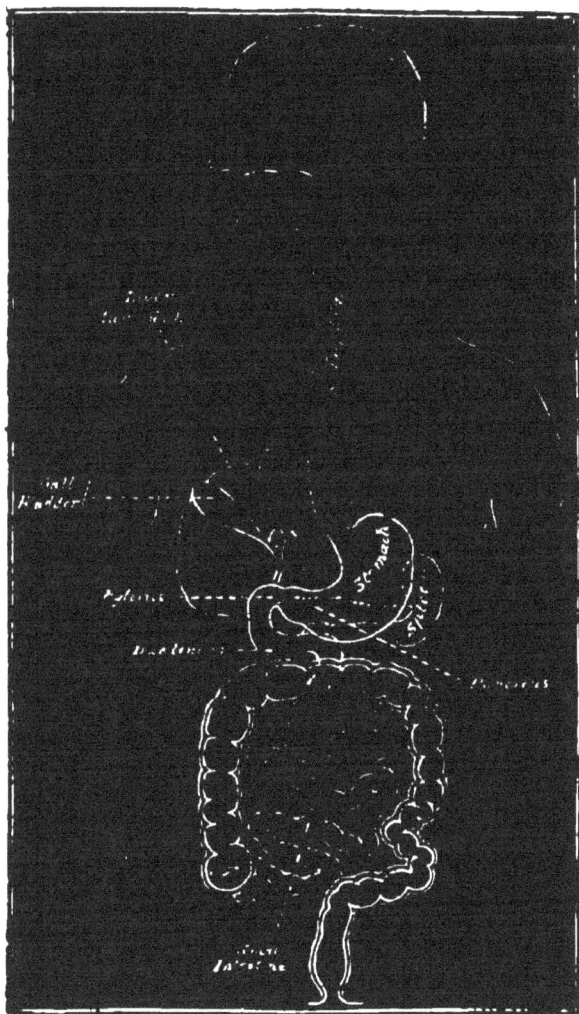

FIG. 33. — Blackboard Diagram of the Digestive Canal.

have a keen appetite for his food, and enjoy it. Young,
growing, and vigorous persons should eat slowly, and
until the appetite is fully satisfied.

It is easy to know when we are eating too much. An overloaded stomach makes itself known by a sense of fulness, uneasiness, drowsiness after meals, and sometimes a real distress. If we keep on eating too much and too rich food, as growing children are apt to do, the complexion becomes muddy, the face marred with blotches and pimples, the breath has an unpleasant odor, and the general look of the countenance is dull and unwholesome.

60. What to eat. — Food should be both nutritious and digestible. It is nutritious in proportion to its capacity to furnish suitable substances to be taken into the blood. It is digestible according to the ease with which it is acted upon by the digestive fluids. Certain vegetable foods are both nutritious and digestible. A man will grow strong and keep healthy on any of them.

The splendid races of Northern India live on barley, wheat, millet, and rice as their staple food. In Southern India, millions of people live on pease and rice. Many generations of the hardiest men in the world, in the north of England and Scotland, have lived on oatmeal and milk. The Roman gladiator was trained on barley ; and the Roman soldier endured his long marches and severe fighting on grain boiled in water, when meat could not be had.

We may safely eat some animal food every day, yet the vegetable albumens supply all that is needed for the nourishment of the body. Solomon briefly puts an important lesson upon this point : " Excess of meats bringeth sickness."

William Cullen Bryant, one of the hardest literary

workers of our times, died at the age of eighty-four from an accident. His breakfast was made of hominy and milk, with a little fruit. He ate meat only once a day. For supper, no tea, but bread, butter, and fruit. Yet when he was over eighty he could do more literary work on this simple diet than most ordinary men of middle age.

Beef, pork, ham, oysters, and rich pastry should be given sparingly to young people. The plainest and simplest diet is the best. It is much better for a child, or any one in fact, to go to bed on a supper of oatmeal, baked apples, or mush and milk, than of hot biscuit, cake, pie, and fried meat; better to begin a day's work with a breakfast of oatmeal, stale bread, a soft-boiled egg, and a glass of milk, than of strong coffee, sausage, and hot bread. Frying food is the worst possible mode of cooking it, and should never be done when it can be avoided.

Some persons are made sick by eating certain articles of food which to most people are harmless. Some are thus affected by various kinds of shell-fish, others by eggs or by fruit. The story is told of a lady who could digest hard salt-beef, but who suffered dreadful pain if she ate a single strawberry; one person was thrown into convulsions whenever he ate onions; Francis the First, a king of France, could not eat bread; and there are several cases recorded of people who had to avoid apples and cheese.

Experience is the only guide for us as to what will disagree with us; and for this reason we have given only hints, not rules, for selecting our daily articles of food.

Eating too frequently, as well as too much at a time, will cause indigestion. The stomach is not an organ intended, as is the heart, to be constantly at work ; after it has done its work, it requires a short period of rest. Most articles of food need from three to five hours to digest.

61. When to eat. — Three meals a day, from five to six hours apart, arranged according to our occupation, should be eaten. The stomach, like other organs, does its work best when its tasks are done at regular periods : hence regularity in eating is of the utmost importance. Eating out of meal-times should be strictly avoided, for it robs the stomach of its needed rest.

Children should not be allowed to eat " between meals." Food eaten when the body and mind are very much fatigued is not well digested. Rest, even for a few minutes, should be taken before a full meal. It is a good plan to lie down, or sit quietly and read, fifteen minutes before eating.

Severe exercise and hard study just after a full meal are very apt to stop digestion. Remember the story of the two hounds. Both were fed alike in the morning. One was taken out on a hunt, the other was tied up at home. When the master came back from the hunt both dogs were killed, and their stomachs examined. It was found that the dog that hunted still had the stomach full of food, while that of the stay-at-home was empty.

The reason is plain : after a full meal, the vital forces of the body are called upon to help the stomach digest the food. If they are forced, instead of this, to help the muscles or brain, digestion is hindered, and a feeling of dulness and heaviness follows. This in time often results in the common form of ill-digestion called "dyspepsia." Healthy persons rarely need food for two or three hours before going to bed. When we are asleep all the vital forces are at a low ebb, and digestion is difficult.

We should make it a point not to skip a meal unless forced to do so. Children, and even grown-up people, often have the bad habit of going to school or to work in a hurry, without eating any breakfast. There is sure to be "an all-gone" feeling at the stomach before another meal-time ; and this, if neglected, is sure, sooner or later, to cause serious injury to the health.

The state of the mind has a great deal to do with digestion, as with the use of every other part of the body. An old Eastern fable tells of a traveller who met the Plague coming from Bagdad.

" You have been making great havoc there," said the man, pointing to the city.

" Not so great," replied the Plague. " I killed only one-third of those who died ; the other two-thirds killed themselves with fright."

Sudden fear or joy, or any startling news, may take away the appetite at once : hence, so far as we can, we should laugh and talk at our meals, and drive away all anxious thoughts and unpleasant topics of discussion. If hunger is a good sauce, so also is a jolly laugh.

62. How to eat. — Eat slowly, and chew the food thoroughly. It is not only bad manners to eat rapidly, but it is a violation of the simplest law of digestion.

Our teeth were made to chew the food, and the saliva to moisten it and help along digestion. If the food is taken slowly, and well chewed, the saliva and the gastric juice act more readily.

Do not take too much drink with the food. If we do so, the flow of the saliva is checked, and digestion is thus hindered. Do not take the food and drink too hot or too cold. Such substances as very hot bread and coffee injure the enamel of the teeth, and are digested but slowly in the stomach. If the food and drink are taken too cold, undue heat is taken from the stomach, and digestion delayed. If we drink freely of ice-water or cold well-water, it will take a long time for the stomach to regain its natural heat.

Drinking freely of very cold water when the body is heated, is also a dangerous practice, and, aside from its ill effects on digestion, has occasionally resulted fatally. It is a poor plan to spur on a flagging appetite with highly spiced food and bitter drinks. An undue amount of pepper, mustard, horse-radish, pickles, fancy meat-dressings, and highly seasoned sauces, may stimulate digestion for the time, but, used in excess, soon weaken it.

63. The Proper Cooking of Food. — The proper cooking and preparation of food is of great importance. It is one of the marked differences between savage and civilized life. It is a serious error to think that the care and labor of the right preparation of food is a degrading work that can be safely left to unskilled, ignorant hands. It requires careful and painstaking intelligence of no mean order.

Whoever is intrusted with this duty for themselves and others should study to secure the variety and method of preparation that the general laws of health demand, and also what is best adapted to individual needs and tastes.

We should not live to eat ; but healthful, well-cooked food, adapted to the physical needs, taste, and power of digestion, of the individual, is one essential to the best kind of life. A neatly set table, with good food, well served, is not only an evidence of civilization, but tends to make us better and happier.

Young women who work in offices, shops, and factories, and know nothing of cooking or other house-keeping duties, should improve the opportunities offered by cooking-schools, or in other ways fit themselves for such duties, before going into homes of their own. All the difference between a well-ordered, happy home and one where disorder and ill-temper rule, is often due to the possession or lack of such knowledge on the part of one who should be the home-keeper.

The man who leaves his home after an unsatisfactory meal of poorly cooked food is far more likely to yield to the temptation to step into a saloon and take a drink than the man who starts out well fed. The alcohol will deaden for a time the uncomfortable feeling that results from the poor food, and thus a bad habit is easily formed of resorting to drinks containing alcohol as a supplement for proper food.

The one whose duty it is to provide, plan, and prepare the meals for a family is often responsible for the habits as well as the health of that family.

64. Care of the Teeth. — We should take the very best care of our teeth, and keep them as long as possible. Teeth are apt to decay. We may inherit poor and soft teeth. Our ways of living may make bad teeth worse. They should be thoroughly cleansed night and morning with a soft brush and warm water. Castile soap, and some simple tooth-powder with no grit in it, may be sometimes used. The brush should be used on the inner or back side of the teeth, as well as on the front side.

It is also very important to clean the spaces between the teeth, and to remove every particle of food ; and that can be best done by passing floss silk between them.

The enamel once broken or destroyed is never renewed ; the tooth is left to decay, slowly but surely : hence we must be on our guard against certain things which hurt the enamel. Picking the teeth with pins and needles is hurtful. We should never crack nuts, crush hard candy, or bite off stout thread, with the teeth.

Dirty and decayed teeth are a frequent cause of an offensive breath and a foul stomach. We should exercise the greatest care to save the teeth. The last resort of all is to lose a tooth by having it taken out. Some one has quaintly remarked, that to lose a grinder is very much like losing an old friend.

65. Effect of Alcohol on Stomach Digestion. — Alcoholic liquors are a mild or a strong irritant of the stomach, just as they are taken raw or diluted, or in small or large quantity. Their habitual use leads to most distressing forms of stomach disease. The color of the inside of a healthy stomach is a deep pink, like the inside of the mouth and throat. Now, if we could look into the stomach, as Dr. Beaumont looked into the stomach of Alexis St. Martin, just after taking raw spirit, we should find that the inner surface would be bright red, far more so than after taking ordinary food. In fact, Dr. Beaumont himself says, that, when Alexis drank brandy and gin, he saw that the inside of his stomach became covered with red patches, and the food he ate was not properly digested.

Alcohol irritates the lining of the stomach, and dilates the tiny blood-vessels, just as brandy dropped into the eye would make it look red and fiery.

Alcohol, like any other irritant, also makes the gastric juice flow ; but it lessens the power of the gastric fluid to digest food, by checking the activity of its pepsin, and at the same time makes some kinds of food more difficult to digest by hardening them.

Now, when this alcohol irritant is poured into the stomach for days, weeks, and even for years, it is no wonder that the stomach becomes altered in its structure. The walls of the stomach become thicker and harder, and after death traces of deep sores are found.

We must remember, that, when the stomach is unable to digest food properly, many other organs of the body suffer as a result.[1]

66. Effect of Alcohol on the Liver. — When alcohol is taken up by the blood-vessels of the stomach, it is carried to the liver, and filtered through this great organ before it reaches the heart. Hence the poisonous effects of alcohol are strongly marked in the liver,

[1] See note 7, page 234.

especially among hard drinkers. The blood-vessels of the liver are overworked, and are engorged with blood.

Many different diseases are produced, some enlarging and others contracting it, but each serious and fatal. A liver which has become contracted from alcoholic liquors is so common, and its cause is so well known, that it is spoken of in every-day language as the " gin-drinker's liver."[1]

67. Effects of Tobacco on Digestion. — Tobacco tends to cause loss of appetite and to weaken the stomach. The smoker sometimes fancies he receives an aid to digestion from his cigar ; but in this he is mistaken. The nerves of his stomach are only paralyzed by the nicotine in the cigar and the indigestion which he has is usually the result of weakening his digestive organs by previous smoking.

In nearly every instance an increase of appetite, a healthier stomach, and a gain in flesh, follow the breaking-off from the tobacco habit.[2]

[1] See note 8, page 235.   [2] See note 9, page 235.

CHAPTER VII

THE BLOOD, THE RIVER OF LIFE

68. The Blood : What it is, How it Looks. — We all know how blood looks to the naked eye. It is a red fluid, which thickens, or clots as it is called, when much of it is shed outside of the body. Let us not be too sure that the blood is red. It is really not red at all, being nearly as colorless as water.

Then, why does it look red ? Let me tell you. The red color is due to millions of little red bodies, called corpuscles, which are swept along in the blood-current like tiny red fishes in the rapids of a river. There are so many of them that they make the blood look uniformly red.

FIG. 34.—Blood Corpuscles.

Fill a clear glass bottle with the smallest red beads, and then with pure water : the water would then look red at a short distance. Imagine the clear waters of a brook alive with little red fishes ; suppose the fishes to be very, very small, and closely crowded together through the whole depth of the stream : the water would look red, would it not ? In a single drop of blood there are about five millions

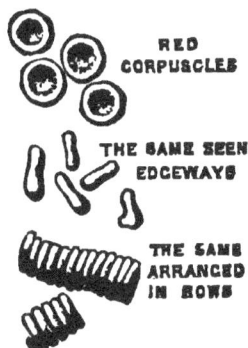

of these bodies ; so you see that they are very tiny
affairs, and very numerous.

If we had fingers delicate enough, we could pack
about fifty thousand of them on the head of a pin.
The shape of these little corpuscles is something like
that of a cent.

Of what use are these red corpuscles ? All the use
in the world. They have the power of taking up gases
as a sponge can take in water. We shall study in the
next chapter something about the oxygen that we
breathe *in*, and the carbonic-acid gas that we breathe
out. Now, these red corpuscles are the oxygen-carriers
for the blood.

We may compare them to a countless fleet of little
boats, carrying their precious cargoes of oxygen to
every part of the body. A very busy life these
corpuscles live. Night and day, whether we are asleep
or awake, these tiny oxygen-carriers are busy as bees.

If we beat up some fresh blood in a bowl with
an egg-beater, we find entangled some white, sticky
threads, which are easily seen after the coloring-matter
has been washed away. This is called **fibrine,** — a kind
of glue used by nature to stop bleeding, by making a
plug for fresh wounds ; otherwise we might bleed to
death from even a slight cut.

Again, if we fill a tumbler half full of fresh blood,
and let it stand over night, we shall find in the morning
it has separated into two parts.

One, a sticky, jelly-like mass, called the **clot,** sinks to
the bottom ; the other, a straw-colored, watery fluid,
called **serum,** is on the top. Serum is made up of albu-

men dissolved in a great deal of water. We cannot boil it. Before we get it as hot as boiling water, it "sets" into a solid mass, like the white of a hard-boiled egg. It is the serum which feeds the tissues of the body with nutritive material.

69. The Circulation of the Blood. — To circulate means to go around, and the circulation is so called because the blood goes round and round in the body. It is carried by a number of pipes, starting from the heart, and branching into all parts of the body.

We know we can draw blood from any part of our bodies if we puncture it with a needle. In fact, there is not a spot on us the size of a needle's point which has not its own little tube filled with blood. Compared with these tiny blood-vessels, our needle is a huge stake, and tears not only one, but a thousand, of these little tubes every time we draw blood with it.

This circulation of the blood has been understood for only about two hundred and fifty years, and the man who made this great discovery richly deserves a few words.

His name was Harvey. He was an Englishman, and a physician to the King of England.

For many years before, learned men had a glimmer of light on the subject; but it was Dr. Harvey who put together all that had been discovered, and really found out the way in which the blood circulates in the human body. The good doctor died in 1657, nearly forty years afterwards; living long enough to see his discovery generally accepted, and himself honored as a benefactor of his race.

70. The Blood-Vessels. — The pipes in which the blood flows *from* the heart are called **arteries,** meaning " air-carriers."

Before the time of Harvey, learned men, not being able to explain the fact that the arteries were found empty after death, supposed that · they carried air, and not blood, throughout the body. The pipes in which the blood flows *toward* the heart are called **veins.**·

Joining these two sets of vessels is another set of little pipes, called **capillaries.** This long name means hair-like, and probably learned men could think of no better way to describe their size than comparing them to hairs ; still, our delicate hairs, fine as they are, are really cables, and coarse cables too, compared to the capillaries. They form a network which serves as a passage-way between the arteries and veins. We may think of an artery and a vein as like two streets, and the capillaries like a host of little lanes through which we must find our way to pass from one street to the other.

Suppose our eyes were sharp enough to watch one of the tiny corpuscles whirling round and round in the circulation of the blood, we should find it sure to get to the heart at last. In brief, the blood-vessels form a sort of ring, — a circle without a break in it. The heart is the centre of the circle.

71. The Heart, the Centre of Circulation. — The **heart** is the most wonderful little pump in the world ; in fact, it is two pumps in one, a double pump. There is no steam-engine half so clever at its work, or so strong.

Most of us know that the heart is in the middle of the chest, between the two lungs, with its pointed end turned towards the left side. Here it is, then, beating like a watch, ticking all day and all night, year after year, never stopping, and never needing to be wound up.

The heart is somewhat like a strawberry in shape, and about the size of the closed fist. It is a muscle, hence it can contract. When it is cut open, it is seen to be hollow inside, and is divided into four rooms. First, it is divided right down the middle from top to bottom ; and there is no door in the partition, so no blood can go from one side to the other. Then, each one of these halves is divided crossways. But this partition is not quite complete : it has little doors that constantly open and shut, which act like the valves of a pump. They open to let the blood through, and close to prevent its return.

Let us now learn the names of these four rooms in the heart, and see what is going on in each. The two upper rooms are called the right and left auricles, the two lower rooms the right and left ventricles. In each, a blood-vessel either enters or starts off.

The largest artery in the body, a big pipe called the **aorta,** goes out of the left ventricle. Did you ever notice a blackish thread running along the backbone of a fish ready for the table ? Well, this is the fish's aorta.

This great tube makes a horseshoe bend near the heart, and, clinging close to the backbone, goes down towards the hips, sending out a great number of branches. Arrived at the loins, it makes a fork dividing into two great branches, which keep on going down, one on each leg, to the very tips of the toes.

Like the trunk of a tree, the arteries divide into branches again and again, and these into still smaller branches and twigs, until at last the capillaries are reached. The countless little capillaries then gradually join together as brooks unite to form a river, and make larger and larger vessels, called veins. By means of these the blood goes back to the heart through the two largest veins in the body, which empty into the right auricle.

72. What takes Place in the Lungs.— How does the blood get from one side of the heart to the other, since there is no opening in that partition which we told you about ? Why, it goes around through the lungs, where it is changed from a dark color to a bright red, or, in other words, is purified by the oxygen of the air.

The blood goes out of the lower room on the right side of the heart by a great tube called the lung artery. This divides over and over again into branches, in the substance of the lungs, until it makes a network of lung capillaries. These unite as they do in the body, and grow into veins which, gradually becoming larger and larger, all unite into four great veins, called lung veins, which empty into the upper room on the left side of the heart. From this side of the heart, the blood is pumped all over the body through the arteries.

Thus the blood goes round and round in the body, making what is called the **circulation;** carrying nutri-

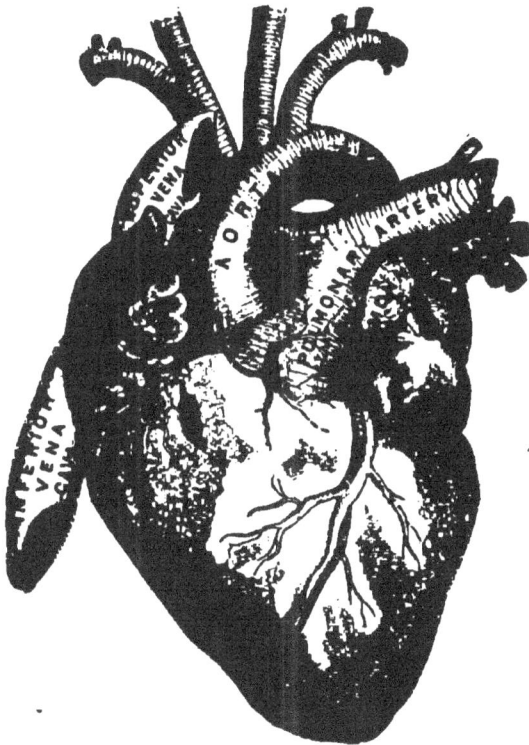

FIG. 35. — The Heart and its Large Blood-Vessels.

ment *to* all the tissues, and bringing away dead matter *from* them.

73. How the Heart does its Work.— The heart is not simply the centre of circulation : it is also the *power* which drives the blood over all the body. It is really a vigorous little force-pump. Every time it beats against our side, it pumps into the arteries a fresh quantity of blood.

The force given by this beat of the heart, added to the elastic pressure of the walls of the vessels, drives the blood through all the arteries, all the capillaries, all the veins, and back again to the other side of the heart.

The heart does this because it is a sturdy muscle, and can draw itself together with wonderful power. If you think for a moment, you will see, that, when the walls of a cavity become at one time shorter and thicker, they draw nearer together, and the space inside becomes very small. This is really what occurs in the four rooms of the heart.

Let us follow a drop of blood in its travels around the body. It returns bright and red from the lungs to the left auricle; this chamber contracts, and the blood is forced down through the trap-door into the left ventricle; then this cavity contracts, and pumps the blood into the aorta; from that forcible impulse, on it rushes through all the arteries, capillaries, and veins, and is at last emptied into the right auricle, a dark, worn-out drop of blood.

This chamber in turn now contracts, and crowds the blood down through the little swinging doors into the right ventricle; this cavity now contracts, and drives the drop of weary blood through the lung artery into the lungs to be purified. Then it is ready once more to go on its restless journey.

More wonderful still! How long do you think it

takes the little drop of blood to go its grand round in the body? Only while you are counting twenty-two. All the blood we have, say about one-tenth of our weight, makes this complete circuit in two minutes.

What a wonderful machine the heart is! It is busily pumping away, without getting tired, night and day, for threescore years and ten, and even a full century, seventy-two strokes every minute, over forty-three hundred times every hour, and nearly thirty-eight million beats every year. Let our heart come to a standstill for one minute, for a second even, and we cease to live.

At each stroke each ventricle pumps about four tablespoonfuls of blood. Nearly seven pounds of blood are moved every minute. How quietly this rapid stream of life flows on within us, never stopping for a second from birth till death! We feel nothing of it but the gentle tapping of the heart, and the regular throb of the pulse, as the life-blood goes on its ceaseless round.

74. **The Pulse, and what it tells Us.** — Press the wrist of a friend, laying three fingers over the outer bone of his arm, or press three of your own fingers over the same bone in your wrist. You can thus feel very easily the **pulse** or beat of the heart, because there is an artery at the wrist, which tells us exactly how the heart is working.

By feeling this, doctors can find out whether the blood is travelling through the body too quickly or too slowly, or just as it ought to do in health. You have probably seen an india-rubber tube on a garden-hose move on the grass at each stroke of the pump-handle. That is a pulse, and is exactly the same as the pulse in our large blood-vessels. The pulse is really everywhere in the body where an artery comes near the surface, as on the temples, the sides of the neck, and near the ankle.

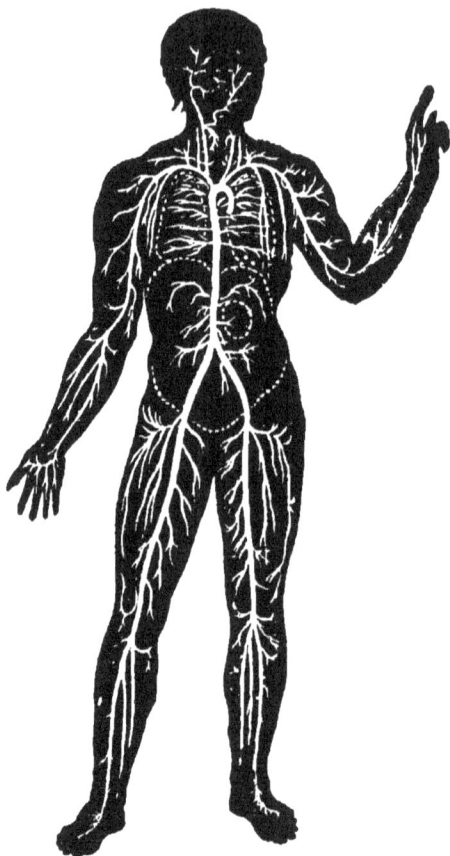

The doctor feels your pulse *at the wrist* simply because it is more convenient for him to do so. Most of the arteries are more deeply buried in the flesh, where it is not easy to reach them.

In a healthy adult, the pulse beats about seventy-two times a minute. In children the pulse is quicker than in adults, and slower in old age than in middle life. Napoleon's heart, it is said, beat only forty strokes a minute. In certain diseases, especially in fevers, the pulse goes with great sudden leaps, like a galloping horse; in others it trots in little jerks; while in a feeble person it moves slowly and

FIG. 36. — Diagram of the Arterial System.

wearily, and its throbs are so weak that we can scarcely feel them.

75. Good Circulation, and how to promote it. — A proper amount of exercise enables all the organs of the body to do their work with more vigor. When we feel cold, a brisk walk or a lively game will "start the blood," make us feel warm. A daily bath, followed by a brisk rubbing of the skin with a coarse towel, promotes the circulation.

Excessive exercise is, however, to be avoided. Like any machine, the heart may be strained by violent efforts. Gymnasts, oarsmen, base-ball players, and others occasionally wrench the delicate machinery of the heart, causing oftentimes many years of ill health.

Many of the veins lie so near the surface of the body, that the flow of blood through them is easily hindered by pressure : hence no article of clothing should be worn tight enough to stop the flow of the blood. Tight garters, by checking the circulation, often cause cold feet and chilblains. Tight collars and clothing about the neck may cause dizziness and a feeling of fulness in the head. Bands, belts, and straps, and even boots and shoes, may be worn tight enough to hinder the free circulation of blood in various parts of the body.

The health of the blood, like that of any other part of the body, may be promoted by a nourishing diet, pure air, and a proper amount of rest and clothing.

76. How Alcohol gets into the Blood. — When one takes an alcoholic liquor into the stomach, some of it at once soaks through the coats of the tiny blood-vessels with which the lining of the stomach is covered, and is carried directly into the blood-current.

Alcohol is also taken up by the lacteals, and is emptied into the blood through the thoracic duct.

It takes only a minute or two for alcohol to get into the main blood-stream. A glass of strong drink soon "goes to the head," as many people know; showing that its effects are rapidly produced in the remotest tissues of the brain.

77. Effect of Alcohol on the Circulation. — In the walls of the blood-vessels are nerves that cause the blood-vessels to contract or expand just enough to keep the right amount of blood flowing through them all the time. When a person takes an alcoholic drink, these nerves are benumbed by the alcohol. They lose their grip on the blood-vessels, which then expand more than they ought, and let too much blood flow through them at one time.

The flushed face of a person who drinks ardent spirits is an every-day sight. It may seem to him and to others a sign of health, but it is really one of the many symptoms of alcoholic poisoning. The alcohol has weakened the nerves which regulate the flow of blood in the vessels. The arteries are relaxed, the capillaries are overflowing, and the undue amount of blood makes the skin look red.

This action we must remember is not confined to the vessels near the surface of the body, but really extends at last to those of every organ and every tissue.

78. Effect of Alcohol upon the Heart. — The heart, like the blood-vessels, is provided with nerves that control its action. One of these may be compared to the balance-wheel of a watch, or the brake on the wheel of a wagon. Remove the balance-wheel or the brake, and the watch ticks wildly, the wagon dashes down the hill at a dangerous rate.

Alcohol deadens this controlling nerve of the heart, and allows it to beat too fast. In addition to this, the nerves having lost their grip on the blood-vessels, the heart has less resistance to overcome. Consequently it is forced to beat faster, and work harder, to fill the dilated vessels with blood. This increased frequency of the heart's stroke means more wear and tear, and less rest ; and this often leads to disease of this vital organ.

With this increased action, there are, to be sure, a flushing of the face, a feeling of warmth, and other marks of increased activity ; but these are not lasting. This effect of alcohol is often called its stimulant action.

But it is in reality the result of its narcotic action, for alcohol has paralyzed the nerves that should control the beating of the heart. Alcohol is not a stimulant, but a **narcotic.** It would be more exact to call these results the beginning of the poisonous effect of alcohol.

79. Effect of Tobacco on the Heart. — Tobacco has a powerful effect upon the action of the heart. A weak and intermittent pulse, due to the irregular action of the heart, is a common result of its use.

This trouble disappears as soon as the tobacco is abandoned. Applicants for life-insurance are frequently rejected because of this trouble, called "a tobacco heart." Dr. Bowditch, one of the most eminent physicians of Boston, considers tobacco nearly as dangerous and deadly as alcohol, and pronounced a man with "a tobacco heart" as badly off as a drunkard.

CHAPTER VIII

HOW AND WHY WE BREATHE

80. What is Breathing ? — Night and day, without one minute's rest, from the first to the last moment of our lives, we are always breathing. About eighteen times every minute, more than twenty-four thousand times every day, we draw in and send out our breath. Most of the time we do not think anything about it. Cats and dogs breathe ; we see their sides move in and out, the same as our chests do. We notice the breath puffing out of a horse's nostrils as he rests after a hard trot. Even plants also breathe, doing it through tiny holes in their leaves, just as truly as animals, though in a different way.

On cold winter mornings we see our breath like a cloud of steam. It feels cold as it passes in over the teeth ; but it is warm as it goes out, for you know we can warm our cold finger-tips with our breath.

Breathing, both by plants and animals, is taking invisible air into the lungs, and sending it out again. Animals breathe by means of a wonderful and beautiful set of machinery, which we will now explain.

◄ **81. The lungs and how they look.** — Strike the upper part of your right chest, just below the collar-bone, with the flat of your hand. Now strike the knee in the same way. See what very different sounds you get.

The lungs lie on each side of your chest, just within the place you struck. The chest sounds quite hollow, about like a drum, because the lungs within it are full of air.

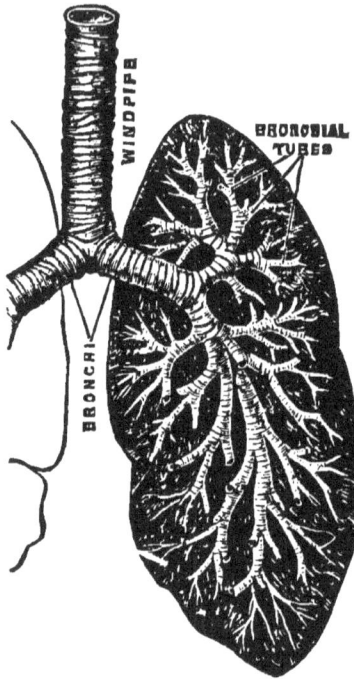

How do the **lungs**, or "lights" as the butchers call them, look? They are two large, pinkish, spongy organs, a mass of air-passages, with arteries, veins, and capillaries, which extend to the collar-bone in front and go down below the shoulder-blade behind.

The next time you go to the market, ask the market-man to show you the lungs, or "lights," of a calf or sheep. Cut off a small piece, and examine it at home carefully. Take a piece in your hand, and you find you have some-thing quite light and soft, which sinks under your finger if you press it, and rises again like a sponge. You will also notice a crackling sound caused by air being forced out of the air-cells.

FIG. 37. — Windpipe and one of the Lungs.

In fact, the lungs, like a sponge, are made up of a countless number of the smallest elastic cavities, into every one of which blood and air keep running, each on its own side, to bid good-day to each other, shake hands as it were, and then hurry out as briskly as they came in.

82. The Air-Passages. — The air is drawn into the lungs through the mouth, nostrils, and windpipe.

The nostrils are really the passage-ways for the air, and warm the air somewhat before it gets into the lungs. If you lean your head back, you can easily feel in the middle of the neck, in front, a stiff tube.

This is the windpipe, which opens into the back of the mouth.

There is a small lid of gristle in front of the open top of the windpipe, which, as you have been told before, is called the epiglottis. It stands upright when we draw air in, and does not in the least prevent the breath from entering the windpipe.

The upper part of the windpipe is a kind of box containing the organs of voice. In this box, easily seen and felt in spare people, and the front of which is commonly called " Adam's apple," are the vocal cords.

These cords are not strings, but elastic strips, with free edges which can be made tight or loose. As the air passes to and from the lungs, through the narrow chink between these cords, it sets them to vibrating, and thus the sound called the voice is produced. During ordinary breathing, the vocal cords are widely separated.

The windpipe runs down through the neck into the chest, dividing into two branches, one going into each lung. It then divides into two others, and

each of these into two more, and so on.   Thus it goes
on dividing into branches, the tubes becoming finer
with every division, until the pipes are smaller than the
tiniest hair.

Every one of these little tubes has on its end a little
hollow ball, called an air-sac, something like a red cur-
rant on its stalk, only much smaller than the smallest
grain of sand.   They are hollow, like tiny bladders ;
and around them, inside,
are little recesses, like
caverns, in their walls :
these are the air-cells.

Imagine a short, thick
tree crowded with leaves ;
imagine the trunk and
all the branches, even
the smallest twigs, to be
hollow.   Suppose the
leaves were tiny blad-
ders, blown up, and fas-
tened to the smallest hollow twigs, and made up
of some delicate but
very elastic substance.
Roughly speaking, so it is with the build of the innermost parts of the lungs.

Around such a framework of hollow branches, called
bronchial tubes, and hollow elastic bladders, called air-
cells, is wrapped a finely woven network of arteries,
veins, and capillaries, like a child's ball covered with a
fine network of red and blue yarn.   As the air fills the

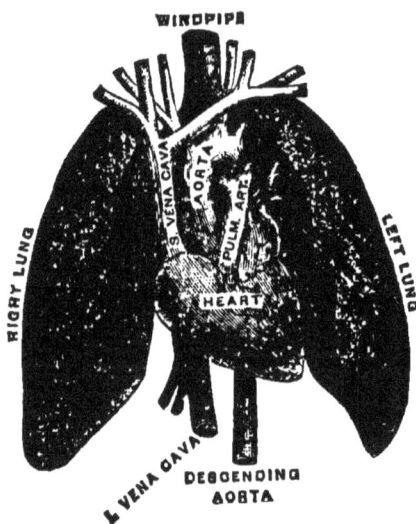

FIG. 38. — The Lungs and Heart
(viewed in front).

elastic cavities in the lungs, just as a boy blows up his toy balloon, the chest swells up ; as the air is forced out, the chest sinks down again.

The whole act of breathing is called **respiration.** Drawing in the breath is called **inspiration;** sending it out is **expiration.**

83. **How we breathe.** — How do we draw our breath ? Let me tell you the simplest things about it. First, the lungs are elastic. The air-tubes and air-sacs make up nearly one-half of the substance of the lung, and nearly the other half consists of blood-vessels. Both the blood-vessels and air-sacs are supported by a framework of elastic tissue.

You know that you can stretch out a piece of elastic to a certain length, and then it springs back to its first size. Just so does this elastic tissue of the lungs act. It is stretched by the air being drawn into the air-tubes, but returns to its first size as soon as the inspiration stops, and so presses on the larger air-tubes, and forces the air out of them.

Second, the lungs are fastened, on the under side, to a great muscle called the diaphragm, which you have already been told about. This is, as you know, stretched like a stout piece of rubber cloth between the chest and abdomen. In its natural position it bulges upwards in the middle, like a handkerchief swollen by the wind, and thus occupies a portion of the chest at the expense of the lungs.

When we breathe air in, its muscular fibres tighten, and make it flat again, just as you make the handkerchief flat by tightening it. When the diaphragm relaxes, the lungs contract, causing their elastic issue to shrink together again ; and so the air is forced out of the larger air-tubes. These up-and-down movements of the diaphragm are the chief movements in ordinary, quiet breathing. This process is repeated over and over again, as long as we live.

This faithful old servant, the diaphragm, quietly began his duties the moment we breathed for the first time. Since that time this sleepless guardian of our life has watched over every breath, and his last effort will be our last sigh. The muscles between the ribs also contract and relax, and are thus useful helps in the act of breathing.

84. What takes Place in the Lungs.— There are two kinds of gas in pure air. The first is very lively and active, called **oxygen.** It is very fond of uniting with other things and burning them. The second gas is a very slow, dull, stupid affair, called **nitrogen;** and nothing will burn in it.

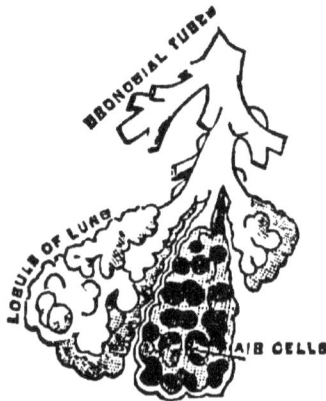

FIG. 39. — The Air-Cells and Bronchial Tubes of the Lungs.

Oxygen, if quite pure, would be altogether too active a gas for us to live in ; so kind Nature dilutes it for us with nitrogen. When the oxygen reaches the tiniest capillaries in the air-sacs of the lungs, it is almost in contact with the blood itself. There is only a very, very thin membrane between the blood and the air.

Now, experiments carried on outside the body prove

that gases can pass through delicate membranes. If a bladder filled with oxygen is hung up in a bottle filled with carbonic-acid, the two gases will mix with each other. The oxygen will pass out through the walls of the bladder, and the carbonic-acid will pass in. This is called the "diffusion of gases."

This is practically what occurs in the lungs. Thus there is an exchange, but no robbery. The red corpuscles of the blood exchange a poisonous gas for one which gives them new life.

We may, in brief, look upon the lungs as a kind of market-place or exchange, where two merchants, the blood and the air, meet to exchange their wares. About twenty cubic inches of air pass in and out of the lungs with every breath, or about what would fill sixty barrels every twenty-four hours. Indeed, it is a very busy market-place.

85. Changes in the Air from Breathing.— When we breathe, we do not simply draw in the air and send it back again. We breathe out some things which were not in the air when we took it in. One of these is water.

On a cold, frosty morning, you know we see the clouds of vapor, or very fine drops of water, coming from our mouths. In hot weather or in a warm room we do not see this vapor, but it is there all the same. If we breathe on a looking-glass, it becomes dim and damp with the water of our breath. There is, of course, a little watery vapor in the air, but hardly any compared to what there is in the breath.

We also breathe out a small amount of animal matter,

—little bits of our own bodies, just ready to decay. This gives the air of an ill-ventilated or over-crowded room the close, disagreeable odor we all know so well. Pure air has no smell.

Again, we send out with every breath a kind of gas called **carbonic-acid gas,** which we can no more see than we can the air itself.

Let me tell you of a simple experiment. Pour some clear lime-water into a goblet. Take a straw, or a sheet of stiff paper rolled into a tube, and blow through it into the lime-water. The carbonic-acid gas of our breath will rapidly make the clear liquid quite milky.

86. How Carbonic-Acid Gas may poison Us. — Carbonic-acid gas in its pure state acts as a deadly poison. If there is too much of it in the air we breathe, it poisons us. We soon breathe hard, get pale, faint, and dizzy, and after a time would die.

Every one has read the story of the " Black Hole of Calcutta." In the year 1756, a cruel tyrant in India, having captured a hundred and forty-six Englishmen, crowded them one hot night into a room where one little window did not admit enough air for the poor prisoners to breathe. They struggled and fought for the air, and in the morning only twenty-three were alive. After one of Napoleon's great battles, three hundred prisoners were crowded into a cave for safe keeping, where in a few hours over two hundred died from the foul air.

In the mines this gas becomes the dreaded "choke-damp." Persons bent on suicide sometimes inhale the carbonic-acid gas from a little charcoal burning in a

closed room. This same deadly gas sometimes flows
naturally from the earth. Some of us have heard of the
" Valley of Poison " in the island of Java. The gas is
very abundant in this valley, and, from its weight, sinks
to the ground, where may be seen, it is said, the skele-
tons of birds and animals which have been suffocated
in their attempt to cross this death-trap.

87. **Pure Air, and how it is kept so.**— One would
think that we should soon use up all the pure air, and
make it all bad. If we think for a moment what a
great number of people there are in the world, — how
many there are in great cities like New York and Phil-
adelphia, — breathing out the carbonic-acid gas from
their lungs, it seems strange there is any air left fit for
us to breathe ; for it is not only men, women, and children who must have oxygen to support their lives, but
also every other animal.

The little worms that live in their holes under ground
want the oxygen of the air just as much as the cows
and the sheep. Even fishes could not live if the water
did not contain air enough for them to breathe.

Why does not the supply of oxygen ever fall short?
What becomes of the carbonic-acid gas ? First, let me
tell you what it is made of : two very good things, —
oxygen and carbon.

A great deal of our flesh and blood is made of these
two things ; but when they are united, and make this
gas, they are of no use to us. We might go to the
store and buy salt and sugar ; but, if they got mixed
together as we brought them home, we could not use
either, unless some good fairy could pick them apart
for us.

Now, can anybody pick apart the carbon and oxygen in the carbonic-acid gas, and make them fit for us to use again? Yes indeed. We have millions of workmen about us that are busily doing this very thing all the time.

Every plant, every green leaf, every blade of grass, does this for us. When the sun shines on them, they pick the carbon out, and send back the oxygen for us to breathe. They keep the carbon, and make that fit for us and other animals to eat. Is not this a wonderful arrangement?

How does all the bad air get out of the towns and cities, where men live, and get to the forests and plains? The wind carries it. Air is constantly moving about, rising up, falling down, sweeping this way or that way, and roving from place to place. In brief, as the Bible tells us, "the wind bloweth where it listeth [pleases]."

88. How People poison Themselves with Bad Air. — Let us now see some other ways in which air may be spoiled, besides by breathing it. Not only the little particles out of our breath, but many other things, may make it unwholesome. Even pleasant odors, like roses or lilies, are unwholesome if shut up in a room.

Dirty walls, ceilings, and floors give the air a musty, close smell ; so do dirty clothes, filthy sinks, and the contents of slop-pails. Some of these ought not to be in the house at all ; others remind us to open our windows wide, and let in pure air.

While all we have told you about pure air applies to persons in health, it applies still more to sick people. First, because sick people need every possible chance to help them get well. They need good air just as much as they do good food. Second, because every thing that comes from a sick person's body is still more unwholesome than that from a healthy person, and may be a downright poison.

Many learned men now believe that numerous diseases are really sown in our bodies by a kind of very small seeds, or "germs," much as plants are sown in the ground. For instance, scarlet-fever, it is claimed, has its own seeds, or germs, which are shed in countless numbers from the body of a person who is suffering from it. Some of these float in the air; and, if we breathe them in, they are quite likely to give us the fever. The same may be true of measles, small-pox, whooping-cough, and other diseases.

Many other things make the air unwholesome. The foul air from chemical works, bone and soap factories, and many other manufacturing places, is more or less hurtful to health. Certain trades shorten life by exposure to air loaded with impurities.

Thus there is the "miner's consumption," due to the dust breathed into the lungs. Those who work on steel, emery, pottery, etc., also breathe in the irritating dust floating in the air. Other impurities are highly injurious to the lungs, as the dust in match-factories, white-lead works, copper and brass founderies, and arsenic in wall-papers.

89. Ventilation, or how to get rid of Impure Air. — How are we to get rid of the bad air in our living-rooms, and to get in fresh air without being too cold? In summer-time this is quiet easy; but in winter it is

more difficult, because it is very uncomfortable and
often dangerous to be cold.   It is a good plan to open
your window at the top, which will let out the bad air.
If you have a good fire and proper clothing, it is very
seldom that you cannot bear the window open a little
way at the top.

Another excellent plan is to raise the lower sash,
putting below it a strip of board two or three inches
wide, the length of the window, and shut the sash on
it.   This leaves at the middle of the window, an opening for fresh air.   If two such windows are thus set on
opposite sides of the room, it gives a constant change
of air, and free from direct draughts.

Good ventilation is just as necessary by night as by
day, because, of course, we go on breathing all night.
People who take pains to shut in the bad and to shut
out the good air, all night long, can never expect to
awake refreshed.

It is very unpleasant to go into the bedrooms of such
people before they have left them in the morning.   It
is not strange that such persons are so often languid,
pale, and peevish all the first part of the day.   We
hardly know why it is people are so afraid of letting in
night air, or what harm it is supposed to do.   Those
who have tried it know very well that they sleep better,
and wake fresher, if they keep the air of their bedrooms clean and sweet all night.   As the famous nurse
Florence Nightingale aptly says, " What other air *can*
we breathe at night ? "

There is hardly a night in the whole year when it is
not safe to keep a window open an inch or two at the

top, and those who do so are not so apt to catch cold as those who do not. We must have, however, proper coverings on our beds to keep us warm.

90. Effects of Alcohol and Tobacco upon the Air-Passages. — Alcohol tends to bring on inflammation of the lung-tissues, and hence to lessen the breathing capacity. The weezy, broken speech of the drunkard is due partly to an irritation of the air-passages, and partly to the thickening of the lung-tissue.

Again, the repeated stretching of the lung capillaries tends to make the habitual user of alcohol more liable to attacks of severe colds and pneumonia ; besides making due allowance for the exposure to cold and wet, so common with the intemperate.

Breathing air full of tobacco-smoke is apt to cause sore throat. The habit of inhaling tobacco-smoke, or breathing it through the nose, is injurious to the throat and lungs. Cigarette-smoke is especially hurtful to the air-passages.[1]

[1] See note 10. page 236.

CHAPTER IX

HOW OUR BODIES ARE COVERED

91. Getting rid of Waste Matters. — When a fire in a stove or furnace burns, it uses up coal and wood, leaving behind dust and ashes ; which must be got rid of, or before long the fire will go out. Our bodies are doing something very similiar. They are all the time useing up our fuel-food, and all the time making some waste matter which must be got rid of.

There are three doors or outlets by which the body rids itself of its waste.

One of these is the **lungs,** which carry off, as we have seen, carbonic-acid gas, water, and animal matter.

The second is the **kidneys,** which filter off water holding a number of salts dissolved in it. The action of the kidneys is explained in more advanced books.

Let us now see how the third outlet of the body, or the **skin,** helps rid the body of its waste matter.

92. How the Skin looks. — Our body is covered with a soft, elastic, tight-fitting garment, — the **skin.** It is easily kept clean, and never wears out. Every child knows how to run a fine needle through the outer skin without feeling it or drawing blood ; but push the needle in a little deeper, and the blood will run at once. Why is this ? Simply because there is a lower, thick layer, full of the finest blood-vessels and nerves, called the **true skin.** The puncture of a pin, or the sting of the tiniest insect, causes pain.

We all know how very tender and painful is the delicate pink skin seen when the outer layer of the blister is torn away. This is the true skin. When it

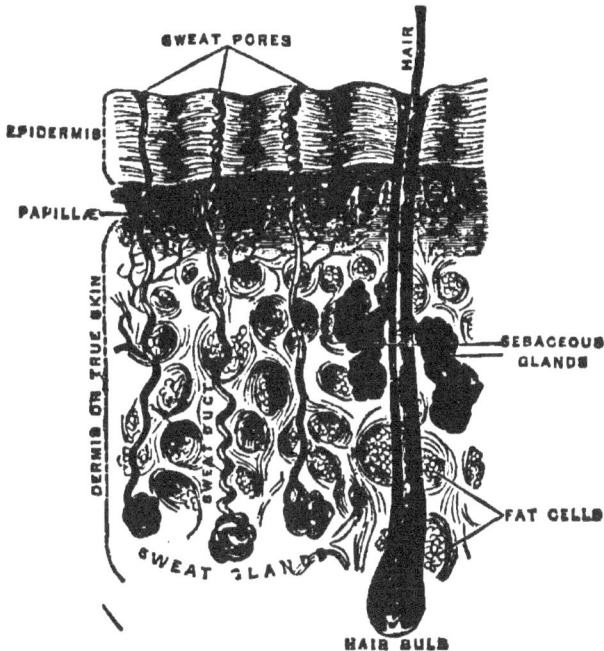

FIG 40. — Vertical Section of the Skin.

is destroyed, a scar results. Look and see if you can find a white scar on your hand, due to a deep cut.

Over the true skin lies another layer of flat, horny, and lifeless scales, in which are no blood-vessels and no nerves. This is called the **scarf-skin,** or **epidermis.** We often give ourselves a little scratch, or pare a corn, without making the blood run, or feeling any pain. It is the scarf-skin which is raised into a blister when we burn our fingers.

The scarf-skin really consists of a countless number of little horny scales, laid one above another, as you might imagine the roof of a house would look with a dozen or more layers of shingles. The outer scales are all the time wearing off and rubbing off, and new ones are always forming underneath.

A snake, as you may know, sheds its whole skin at once, as if a boy should crawl out of his clothes ; and sometimes you may find in the fields its cast-off skin turned inside out, just as the snake squirmed out of it and crawled off with a soft new dress on. Now, we shed our skin a little at a time, and in such tiny, powdery scales that we cannot usually see them.

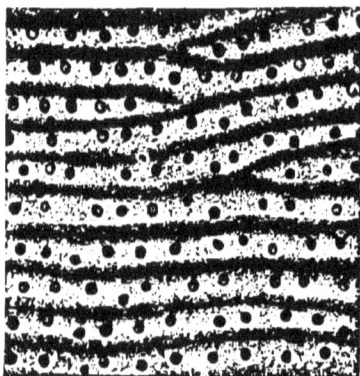

Fig 41. — The Scarf-Skin from the Palm of the Hand, showing the Pores.

If we take any garment that has been worn next the skin, and shake it in the sunlight, we see how much dust there is inside of it. This dust is really little bits of the scarf-skin which have dropped off or worn away. Where the skin is pretty thick, as on the palms of the hands or the soles of the feet, we can, when we wash ourselves, see dead skin peeling off in little scales.

93. **The Sweat : what it is, and where it comes from**. — If we look at the skin on the tip of the fingers

through an ordinary magnifying-glass, we see a great number of little holes called pores. Just think how small they are ! More than five thousand have been counted on the tip of one finger, and there are more than three millions of them in the covering of the whole body.

Each pore is the end or opening of a tube called a sweat-gland. Each gland is a tiny tube just under the scarf-skin, rolled round and round like a ball of the finest silk. If all the sweat-glands in our body could be unrolled, and laid end to end like a long gas-pipe, they would be about four miles long.

What work do these sweat-glands do ? Why, a great deal of it. Let me tell you about it. Certain waste matter picked up by the blood is strained out through the thin walls of the blood-vessels into the sweat-glands, up which it rises until it runs out of the openings, when it is called **sweat.**

If we hold the tip of our finger very close to a mirror, but without touching the glass, we see the place has become dim and moist. This is because the sweat has oozed out of the pores of our finger on the glass. If the mirror were held to any other part of the skin, it would become dim and moist just the same.

Thus we see that the sweat-glands, if they are kept in good order, serve as little drain-pipes to rid our bodies of waste matters. When the weather is very hot, or when we are working hard, or are exposed to much heat, the sweat flows so freely that it stands on the skin in big drops ; but at other times it flows more slowly.

Still, it is always oozing out, even in the coldest winter weather. About two pints of sweat ooze every day through these busy little glands in the skin.

The skin is naturally soft, and the hair moist and glossy. What makes them so ? Two little **oil glands,** attached to each hair, furnish this natural dressing for the hair and the skin. We may call it Nature's hair-oil.

94. Why we need to wash ourselves. — A great deal of the sweat soaks into our clothing, so that it needs frequent washing ; but most of the moisture dries off into the air, and so cools the body. Some of the oily matter, however, sticks to the skin, and, together with the dirt or dust from the outside, makes a little plug, as it were, over the pores. The waste matter cannot filter through the skin, and has to stay in the body, or find its way out elsewhere.

Suppose the drain-pipes which lead from a house should get stopped up ; we can imagine what an unhealthy state the house would soon be in. Just so it is in our body if the little pipes which drain the skin get clogged. If a person had his skin varnished all over, so as to stop up all the pores, he would die within a few hours.

An instance proving this occurred at Rome many years ago, when the body of a little boy was completely covered with gold-leaf, in order that he might play the part of a cherub or an angel in a show. He was afterwards put to bed without the gold having been washed off ; and, when his parents tried to rouse him the next morning, he was dead.

It is said that the reason why the small-pox was so

fatal among the Indians in this country was because they always kept the pores of their skin closed with bear's grease, to protect them against cold, and daubed themselves with earthy paints for the sake of ornament.

How necessary, then, it is to have a clean skin, and to wear clean clothes! Many people think they have done quite enough if they wash every day their hands and faces, and the parts that are seen; but it is even more necessary to wash the parts of the body that are not seen, and are covered with our clothes, because all the dirt which comes from inside the body stays on the surface, and is not rubbed off, as it might be on our hands or faces.

95. The Hair and the Nails. — The hair and the nails really belong to the skin.

The hair grows out from little sacs or bags in the skin, and so do the nails. Every hair has a little bulb or root, which is fixed in the skin, and soaks up the nourishment from the blood-vessels.

It adds to our health and comfort to keep the hair clean. The oil-glands get clogged; and the dust and dirt, rapidly making a coating, commonly called "dandruff," on the scalp, get caught in the hair. Hence the hair should be often washed, combed, and brushed.

The color of the hair is given to it by little bags filled with coloring-matter. These are found in the hair and in the skin. In some people, especially old persons, this, Nature's paint-stuff, dries up; and the hair becomes colorless, or, as we say, begins to turn gray. When Nature spatters some extra drops of her paint here and there, especially on the face and arms, we call them freckles. Sudden fright or great sorrow will sometimes turn the hair white in the course of a few hours.

It is said, that, at the time of the cruel Revolution in France, the hair of the poor French queen, Marie Antoinette, turned white in a single night, owing to the distress and agony of mind she suffered for the safety of her husband and her children.

The nails of our fingers and toes grow out from our skin, like broad, flat hairs and are really only a kind of horny skin. They serve to protect the ends of the fingers and toes. Some people, especially school-children, spoil the look of their fingers by biting their nails : so that, instead of pretty oval, bright-pink, shell-like ornaments, as they should be, we see only ugly, stumpy fingers, with sore tips to them, which can feel nothing delicately or tenderly.

The toe-nails require as much attention as the fingers. If we look at a baby's tiny foot before it has worn shoes, we see how pretty the little toes and nails are.

The finger-nails should be trimmed with scissors once a week, leaving them long enough to protect the ends of the fingers. Nails should never be trimmed to the quick. They should not be cleaned with any thing harder than a brush or bit of soft wood. They should not be scraped with a penknife or scissors, as these hurt their nice polish. To prevent hangnails, the skin should be often loosened from the nail, not with a knife or scissors, but with something blunt, such as the handle of a tooth-brush, or an ivory paper-cutter.

96. Baths, and how to take them. — It takes very little time, expense, or trouble to take a daily bath of some sort. A hand-basin, a sponge, a strip of cotton-flannel, a piece of castile-soap, a gallon of water, and a towel, are all that are required.

Even rubbing the body every day, first with a damp towel, and afterwards very briskly with a dry one, will in most cases keep the skin clean enough during the week, provided a bath with soap and warm water is taken once a week. Most persons, especially the young and vigorous, soon get used to cool, and even cold, water baths.

The first effect of any cold bath is to shrivel up all the vessels of the skin, and make it look like "goose-flesh." Brisk rubbing will soon cause a glow, or bring on a re-action as it is called, after which a feeling of genial warmth is felt all over the person. Coarse towels should always be used if the skin will bear it.

It is a good time for vigorous persons to take a cold bath just after getting out of bed in the morning. A bath at bedtime is refreshing, and favors sound sleep. There is little risk of taking cold if we go to bed at once. Young and feeble children should bathe two or three hours after breakfast.

Swimming in running fresh water or in the salt water has a wholesome effect on the skin, and is one of the healthiest of all exercises. So highly did the Romans regard this art, that, to express their contempt for an ignorant person, they would say, "He can neither read nor swim." Young people should be taught to practise it whenever it is convenient.

Never go in swimming when the body is over-heated or very tired. Better sit down quietly, and cool off for half an hour. Many are drowned every year from ignorance or carelessness in this matter alone. The risk is from sudden cramps, which cause even a strong swimmer to sink like a lump of lead. For the same reason, it is not safe to take a swim just after a full meal. Alexander the Great once nearly lost his life by swimming in a very cold river just after a meal.

Thirst may be relieved by bathing the body in water, and medicines have been taken through the skin. Poisons may also be absorbed by the skin. For this reason, alcohol should not be used for bathing purposes, as it may thus be taken up by the skin into the blood. Common salt, or preparations known as sea salt, are far better to use with the bath.

97. **Why the Body is warm.** — Every one knows that the outside of the body is warm. If we get into a cold bed on a winter's night, our body soon warms it, and, however cold we feel at first, the heat of our bodies, like a fire always burning, keeps up the warmth of the bed.

Put a little thermometer in your mouth, and close the lips around it for five minutes. What do we find? Why, on taking out the instrument, we find that the natural heat of the body is about ninety-eight degrees Fahrenheit, even on the coldest day of winter or the hottest day of summer.

Where does this heat come from? How does the body make this heat? Let me try to help you understand this by reminding you of what you have already been told about air in a preceding chapter.

Oxygen is, as we know, very fond of joining itself with other things, and burning them. When oxygen joins itself with any other thing, it always makes some heat ; and it is called a burning, whether there is any flame or not.

We know that we are in some ways very much like a candle. Let me tell you of another way. When a candle is burning, what really takes place is, that the different things of which the candle is made unite with the oxygen to make carbonic-acid gas.

There is another gas in the candle, called hydrogen, which unites with the oxygen to turn into water. This goes on very fast indeed, and makes the candle very hot. Now, we know there is plenty of carbon in our bodies, and also plenty of hydrogen. When the oxygen of the air comes near them, they unite with it, and burn, as a candle does, and turn into carbonic-acid gas and water. This makes us warm.

The great difference is, that they do not burn nearly as fast in our bodies as they do in the candle ; therefore we do not flame and blaze up, nor are we nearly so hot as a lighted candle. A piece of fat, for instance, burns rapidly and brightly when put in the fire.

But, if we eat the piece of fat, it will make just as much heat within our bodies as if we burned it in the fire. True, the burning will not be so rapid, nor the degree of heat produced so great ; but it will last for a much longer time, and the total quantity of heat given out will be the same in both cases.

Hence our bodies are warm because we are burning away bit by bit, just as a candle does. Every time we

move, feel, think, or, in fact, do anything at all, this
burning goes on. Thus our bodily heat is produced,
and life is kept up.

In brief, Nature warms our bodies on somewhat the
same plan by which we warm our houses with a coal-
stove in the winter.

98. How the Heat of the Body is regulated.—
How is it that the warmth of the body is the same at
every season of the year and in every climate? Let me
try to make this plain.

If we put a drop of water, ether, or alcohol on the
back of our hand, we feel the skin there grow colder;
this is because the heat required to evaporate the liquid
is taken from the skin. As the sweat evaporates from
our skin, it produces cold. Now, the hotter the air outside of us, the more we sweat ; but, as fast as the sweat
comes out of the pores, it evaporates, and so more cold
is produced.

In this way the heat of the skin and of the blood is
kept from rising much above ninety-eight degrees
Fahrenheit. If the air outside is very cold, the pores
contract, and very little sweat comes out of them.

Thus, in summer and in hot countries the abundant
sweating tends to cool our bodies ; while in winter and
in cold countries, since little sweating takes place, the
body does not lose much heat.

Men who have to work in the midst of great hot
furnaces, such as blacksmiths or workers in iron-found-
eries and glass-works, are no hotter inside their bodies
than fishermen or teamsters. The blood may become
hotter or colder from causes within us, — for instance,

fevers make it hotter; want of food makes it colder, — but it has such a power of resisting the heat and cold outside the body, that persons have been known to go for a few minutes into ovens hot enough to bake bread.

Years ago there was a man, called the "Fire King," who could go into a red-hot oven, and stay five minutes. It was found, while he was in the oven, that the heat of his blood was exactly the same as when he entered it. We may be sure that he sweated profusely.

It is because the blood always keeps at about the same degree of warmth, whatever the heat or cold outside, that people are able to live in all climates, and to bear all seasons.

The Esquimau, who lives amidst the ice and snow of polar regions, has as much warmth in his blood as the African, who lives under the scorching sun of the tropics. Man is the only animal that endures and flourishes in every climate of the globe.

99. **Why we need Clothing.** — A thin and delicate skin is our only covering. Why do we need any other? Why do we need clothing? Let me tell you.

Our bodies are, as you know, much warmer than the air out of doors, so they are continually giving out their heat to the air. When our bare skin is exposed, we lose heat rapidly, and feel chilly and cold : hence we wear clothes to keep the heat of our bodies from escaping too rapidly into the air.

Is there another reason? Yes. In hot summer weather, especially in hot countries, the direct rays of the sun would scorch our skin. Again, clothes save the skin from being torn or hurt by accidents. They also keep out the wet, so that we can better bear exposure to rain or snow. The frequent changes of weather, so common in this country, are a severe tax on the body, against which our clothes are our chief means of defence.

100. Hints about wearing Clothes. — Clothes should be changed according to the climate or season of the year. It is not prudent to leave off winter clothing too early in the spring, for our seasons are most uncertain. Woollen clothing should be worn next to the skin, whether in summer or winter.

A most imprudent but common error is to take off our winter flannels early in summer because it happens to be warm. With our sudden changes of weather, a person may thus run great risk of taking severe colds, pneumonia, and even "quick consumption."

A wise doctor has said, " Never allow yourself to feel cold. Whenever you feel chilly put on more clothing, go into a warmer room, or exercise. In some way get warm and keep warm. Only beggars and fools go cold. The former, because they lack clothes ; the latter, because they do not know enough to wear them."

To keep our persons neat and clean, we must change our clothes often. This applies not only to garments used for daily wear, but to bed-clothes and night-clothes. No one should sleep in the clothes he wears during the day. Undergarments should be frequently and regularly changed. Bed-clothes should be exposed freely to the light and air.

Young children are less able than grown-up people to

resist cold and sudden changes, hence great' care must be taken as to their clothing. The legs and chests of children should not be exposed to the bitter blasts of winter nor to the cold winds of spring. Hundreds of children die every year from diseases due to ignorance or neglect in this matter.

Never wear wet or damp clothes one moment longer than possible. Little harm results from wearing wet clothes, provided the person keeps actively moving about while they are drying on him. If you have on wet clothes, take the shortest way home, rub down thoroughly, and put on at once dry warm clothes. Do not let your damp skirts, wet stockings, or shoes dry on you ; but always change them at once.

Do not wear clothing tight enough to prevent the free movements of the body. See to it that children wear proper outside garments on going out, and that they are taken off on coming in-doors. Pupils should not sit in the schoolroom with outside garments on, such as water-proofs, gossamers, cloaks, rubbers, rubber boots, and leggings.

101. **Alcohol and the Bodily Heat.** — Soon after taking a small quantity of alcohol, there is a feeling of warmth over the surface of the body. The body is not really warmer, but the skin feels warmer. On the contrary, we are really colder, because heat is more rapidly lost from the surface. The skin is warmer after taking alcoholic liquor, because the nerves that regulate the hair-like vessels on the surface, being weakened, lose their grip : hence more blood is sent at first from the inner parts of the body to the surface.

There is no real increase of heat ; the surface is warmed for the time, at the expense of the deeper portions of the body. This surface warmth is now rapidly lost, and the general heat of the body is lowered below its natural temperature.

Experience has proved, time and time again, that alcohol lessens our power to endure extremes of heat and cold. Arctic explorers find that exposure to severe cold can be endured far better without alcohol. Whoever takes an alcoholic liquor to help him bear the cold makes a great mistake. Such a drink, as we have seen, will reduce the heat of his body, cause him to suffer more, make him more liable to take cold, and to freeze if long exposed.[1]

Army life is, perhaps, the best possible test. It is the almost universal experience of British army officers who have led their men through the campaigns in the hottest parts of India and Africa, that alcohol, so far from being a help to resist great extremes of heat, acts as a positive injury.

The skin depends for its nourishment upon the proper circulation of the blood in the blood-vessels. When this is interfered with by alcohol the skin is not properly nourished. Dark brown blotches appear. The blood-vessels of the face become permanently stretched and can be distinctly seen underneath the skin, while the red and swollen nose is so marked a result of alcohol-poisoning that even children know it by a familiar nickname.

102. **Effect of Tobacco upon the Skin.** — Tobacco gives the skin a peculiar dry and sallow look. If a

---

[1] See note 11, page 237.

confirmed tobacco-user be put in a warm bath the odor of the tobacco will be very easily perceived in the room when he comes out, while a fly dropped into the water in which he has bathed will be quickly killed.

This shows how even the pores of the skin of the tobacco-user become saturated with the poison. But we need not put him in a bath to discover this. The tobacco essence is constantly passing out of his skin through his clothes until they become so filled with it that we can smell it as we pass him on the street.

The smoker, however, is entirely unconscious of this. His senses are so blunted that he fails to notice the odors that make him offensive to all the cleanly people he comes near.

.

CHAPTER X

THE NERVOUS SYSTEM: HOW IT GOVERNS THE BODY

103. **How all parts of the Body work together for its good.** — We have studied the human body as a kind of living machine. We have examined its various parts, and found each adapted, not only to take care of itself, but to do some special work essential to the well-being of the whole.

Everywhere organs are working together for the common good. Strike suddenly at the eye, and the lids shut to protect it. Tickle the foot, and the muscles of the leg pull it away.

Fifty skilled mechanics might do their best at building a house ; but, if each worked as he pleased, the result of their work would be of little value. The master-builder must be at his post, skilful to direct, and quick to act. So with our bodies ; and the wonderful agency which governs every part of our bodies is the nervous system.

Let us learn a few things about its several parts, the brain, the spinal cord, and the nerves.

104. **The Brain.** — The brain is one of the most wonderful and important organs in the body. It fills the inside of the skull, and is a curious, pulpy-looking mass, not unlike blanc-mange. The outer surface is

grooved into folds something like the appearance of a crumpled silk handkerchief.

The brain consists of two parts, — one large, the other small. The upper portion, or brain proper, is

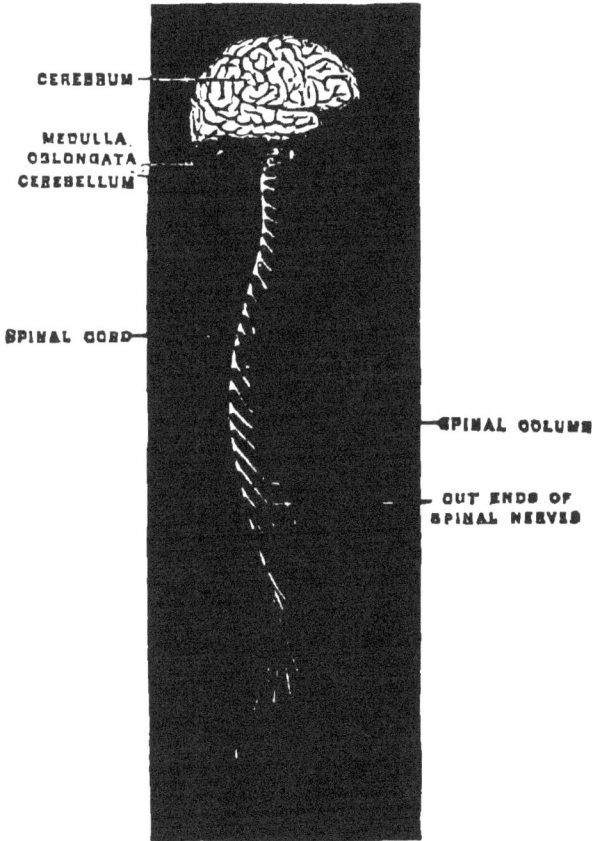

CEREBRUM

MEDULLA
OBLONGATA
CEREBELLUM

SPINAL CORD

SPINAL COLUMN

OUT ENDS OF
SPINAL NERVES

FIG. 42. — Diagram of Brain and Spinal Cord.

nearly seven-eighths of the whole mass. It is in halves, one on each side, separated from each other by a deep groove. The little brain lies beneath the back part of the brain proper.

How much do you suppose the brain weighs? Well, about three pounds.   As   a   rule,   a   large   brain   is the sign of a superior mind. Daniel Webster's brain weighed fifty-three and a half ounces. Agassiz's weighed the same.   That of Cuvier, the celebrated natural-ist, weighed sixty-four ounces and a third.   An idiot's brain rarely ex-ceeds thirty ounces.

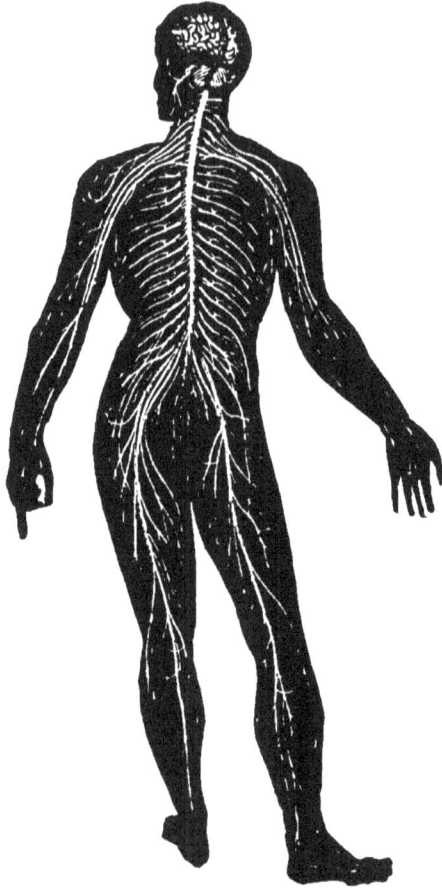

105. The Nerves. — Now, our backbone, or spine, has inside of it a large nerve, about two feet long, of a whitish-gray color, called the **spinal cord.**   This goes from the brain down the back of the neck ; and all along it gives out little white, glis-tening threads, called **spinal nerves.**   These come off in pairs from the spine, one to each side of the body ; sending out many other branches as they go.

Fig. 43. — Diagram of the Brain, Spinal Cord, and Nerves, from behind.

These nerve-branches go to the muscles, to the organs, to the skin, and to the tissues generally.   In fact, every part of the body you could touch has nerves in it.

If you could follow a nerve along its course, you would find, by and by, that you trace it into either the

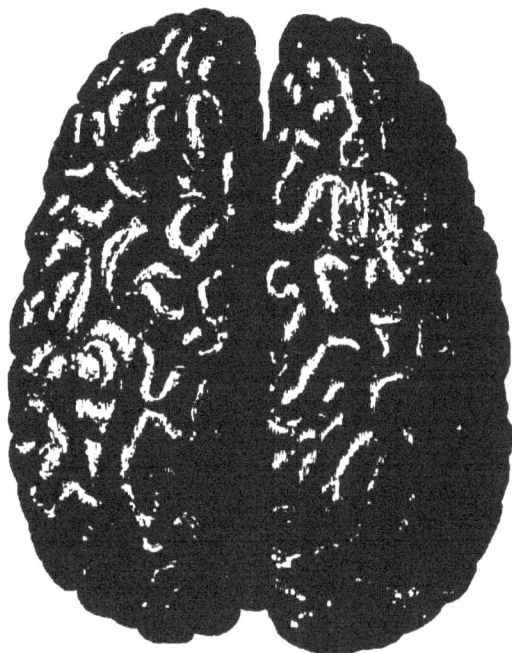

FIG 44. — Upper Surface of Brain, showing the Convolutions and its Double Structure.

spinal cord or the brain itself, — most likely into the cord, for the greater number of the nerves of the body branch out from it.

Now, messages pass along these nerves *from* the brain, and also back *to* it It is in the brain that we feel and will. No part of the body has in itself any feeling, or any power of willing its own movement. If all the nerves leading from your hand to the brain were

cut across, you would not feel any pain in your hand,
nor could you move it at all.

106. The Telegraph System in our Bodies. — The
nervous system is like a complete telegraphic system.
The brain is the main office ; and the thousands of
nerve fibres, branching off to all parts of the body, are
the telegraph-wires. Despatches are constantly being
sent to the brain, to tell what is going on in various
parts of the body. The brain, on receiving the news,
at once sends back its orders as to what must be done ;
and the order flies through the nerves faster than it is
possible for us to think.

Thus, if you put your hand accidentally on a hot
stove, you would not be long in pulling it away. Yet
really this is what happened : a message flashed along
the nerves from your hand, through the spinal cord,
to the brain, "We are burnt !" The brain at once
returned the message to the muscles, "Pull the hand
away !" Then the muscles contracted, and the hand
was removed.

107. What is meant by Reflex Action. — Now,
every message from various parts of the body does not
travel as far as the main office, — that is to the brain, —
but some of them are switched off, or "reflected" as
we call it, at some of the little offices on the way.

These way-stations, located along the spinal cord,
receive messages, and send back answers, without con-
sulting the brain. If some one should tickle our toes
when we were 'fast asleep, we would draw our feet
away ; and yet we would know nothing about it when
we awoke.

In eating we sometimes get a crumb into the windpipe, and cough hard to get rid of it. We cannot help
coughing : it goes on without our will. This is called a
reflex action. The impressions made by the tickling
and the crumb do not go to the brain ; but the signal
of danger or distress is sent to one of the way-stations
in the cord, and the order to do something is sent back,
or "reflected" to the muscles which control the part in
need of help.

108. **The Importance of Reflex Action.** — Did you
ever think how important reflex action is to our health,
comfort, and safety ? Ten thousand acts take place
which tend to keep us well, and yet we have as little
control over them as over the stars above us. If the
feet slip, the body tends to recover itself without the
effort of the will. We try to brush the flies away when
we are asleep.

The story is told of an old soldier who, while carrying
a bowl of soup across the street, suddenly dropped it on
hearing some wag call "Attention !" so used was he,
at that word of command, to stand erect with his hands
at his side. By an effort of the will, we can stop our
breath for a moment or two ; but soon the call for air
must be obeyed, whether we will or not. The great
work of digestion is going on all our lives, and we have
no control over its complicated movements.

What is the good of all this ? Why, all the good in
the world. By this wonderful provision, our brain is
relieved of a vast amount of work. If we were forced
to use our will-power to digest our food, the brain would
be put to a constant strain. We could not, as now, eat

and then go about our business.   If we had to plan and
will every heart-beat, we should soon be tired of life.
We could never sleep ; for the brain would be on the

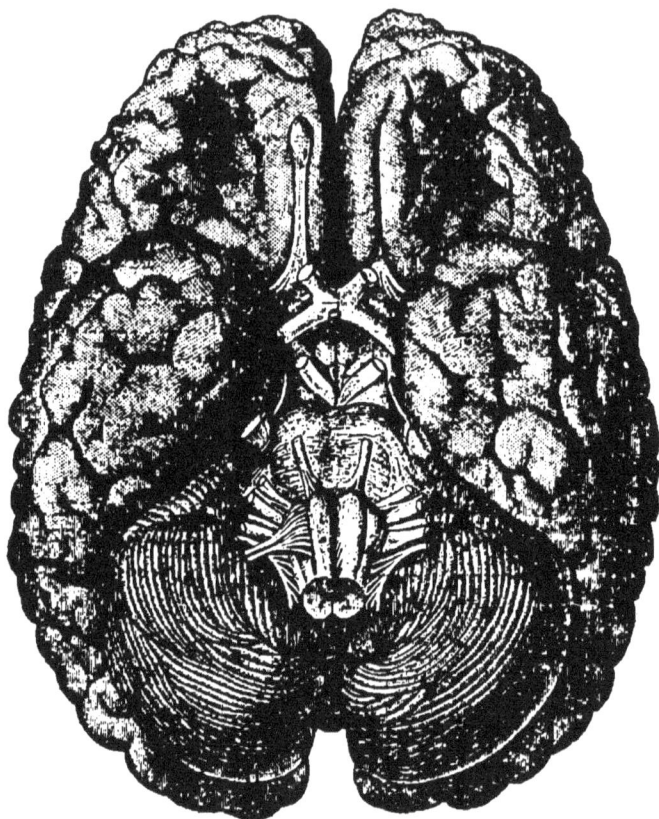

FIG. 45.— Under Surface of the Brain.

watch to decide if it were time for the next heart-beat,
the next breath, and the proper time for each digestive
fluid to flow.

109. The Health of the Nervous System. — The
health of the nervous system is woven into the welfare
of every organ in the body, just as colored threads are

woven through a piece of cloth.   An injury to one part
affects another part, through the shock to the nervous
system.   A blow on the head often causes vomiting.
An overloaded stomach may make the brain dull and
stupid for several hours.   Ill digestion may make us at
times cross and peevish.

Let a small artery inside the skull be broken by a
fall or a blow, and a clot no larger than a bean may be
formed, which presses on the brain ; and complete loss
of motion on one side may result.   An accidental blow
on the head gave a European ruler, a man of limited
intellect, ever afterwards a wonderful memory.   It is not
an uncommon thing for a person to fall and strike his
head, and thus produce a fatal disease of the kidneys.

The brain, or the thinking-part, is a most precious
gift.   It needs exercise, as well as any other organ.
As its office is to think, we should give it good things
to think about, just as we give the stomach good food
to digest. . How necessary it is to keep it sound and
healthy !

We should bring the brain into the habit of thinking
in earnest, so that it may grow strong and vigorous.   A
gentleman once asked a boy who was idling about the
fields, " What are you thinking about ? " — " Mostly
naught, sir," said the boy ; and so it would be with many
young people if they were left to themselves, and not
taught from their infancy to think.

The little brain of a child should be trained to all
that is true, noble, and good.   Children should be
encouraged to find out all they can about flowers, birds,
trees, and animals, and to learn all about this beautiful

world.   We must learn to use our reason and judgment in all that we do.   Self-indulgence should be the
last object we have in mind.   Self-control is one of
the greatest victories we can gain in life, and it will
help us to many more.

Unhealthy and evil habits are steady drains upon the
limited amount of nervous force that each one has.   All
forms of sensual gratification that excite pleasure, only
to be followed by depression, cause a great waste of
nervous energy, and tend to sap the very foundation of
health and happiness.

110. **Sleep, and how to get it.** — Of all the wonderful
things about us which we do not wonder at because
they are so common, sleep is one of the strangest.
How it comes, why it comes, how it does its kind,
helpful work, not even the wisest people are able to
tell.   We do not have much trouble in seeking it : it
comes to us of itself.   It takes us in its kindly arms,
quiets and comforts us, repairs and refreshes us, and
turns us out in the morning quite like new people.

Sleep is necessary to life and health.   We crave it
as urgently as we do food or drink.   In our waking
hours, rest is obtained only at short intervals : the
muscles and nerves, and the brain are in full activity.
Repair goes on every moment, whether we are awake
or asleep; but during the waking hours the waste of
the tissues is far ahead of the repair, while during sleep
the repair exceeds the waste.   Hence good mother
Nature at regular intervals causes all parts of the
bodily machinery to be run at their lowest rate ; in
other words, we are put to sleep.

Sleep is more or less sound, according to circumstances. Fatigue, if not too great, aids it; while idle-

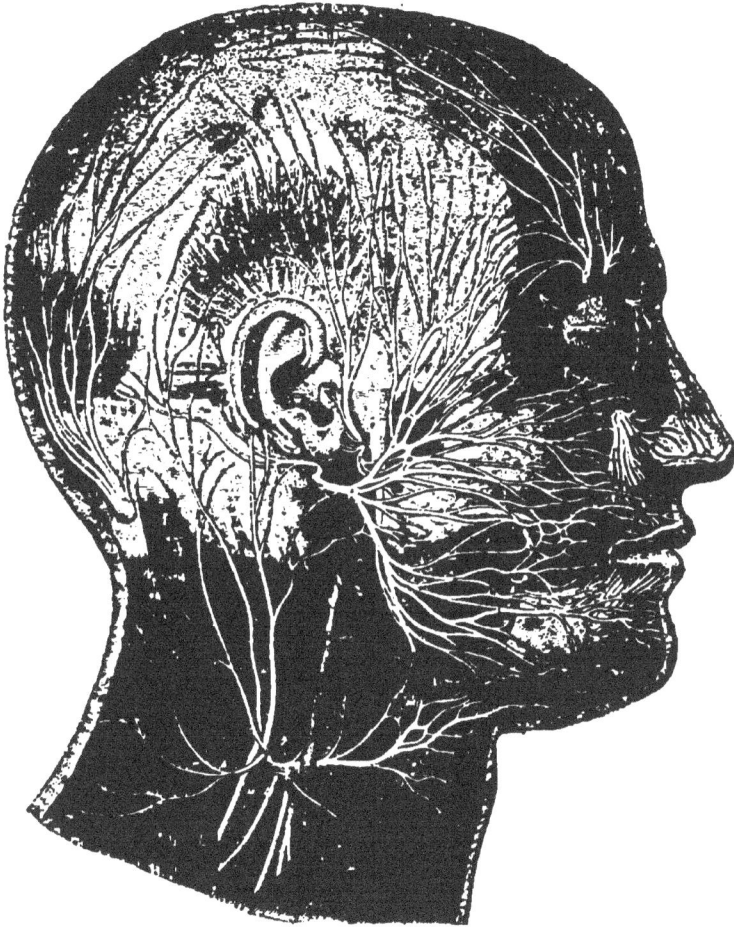

FIG. 46. — Superficial Nerves on the right side of the Neck and Head.

ness lessens it. Some drinks, as tea and coffee, may prevent it. Anxious thought, and pain, and even anticipated pleasure, may keep us awake: hence we should not go to bed with the brain excited or too active. We should read some pleasant book, laugh, talk, sing, or take a brisk walk, or otherwise rest, for half an hour before going to bed.

The best time for sleep is during the silence and darkness of night. People who have to work nights, and to sleep during the day, have a strained and wearied look. The amount of sleep depends upon the temperament of each individual. Some require little sleep, while others need a great deal.

Eight hours of sleep for an adult, and from ten to twelve hours for children and old people, is about the average amount required. Frederick the Great and Napoleon were light sleepers, four hours daily being the usual time given to sleep by these tireless warriors.

Most of the world's great workers have recognized the necessity of a goodly amount of sleep. Sir Walter Scott, the great master of fiction, took much exercise, and always insisted upon having eight hours of sound sleep every night.

Children naturally need more sleep than grown-up people, because their bodies require more rest during the period of growth : hence children should be put to bed early, and sleep in the morning until they awake. Children should not play too hard during the hour before bedtime ; but the time should be spent in quiet and restful talk, avoiding startling stories.

When fairly awake, we should get up. Dozing, neither asleep nor awake, is not healthful, especially for young people. The Duke of Wellington used to say, "When it is time to turn over, it is time to turn out."

111. **Effect of Alcohol on the Nervous System.** — We must remember that alcohol is a narcotic,[1] that it deadens or paralyzes the nerves and the brain of the drinker, if we would understand its effect upon the nervous system.

One of the first results after an alcoholic drink has been taken, is the quickened action of the heart ; but even this is caused by the deadening or benumbing of the nerves that, as we have learned in a previous lesson, should hold the heart in check and not let it beat too fast.

Now we must remember that the brain is very richly supplied with blood-vessels. The nerves in the walls of these blood-vessels that should regulate the flow of the blood are also deadened by the alcohol, and that allows the blood-vessels to stretch too much, and too much blood rushes to the brain. This causes the flushed face and undue excitement. The mind seems for a time to become more active.

Because thoughts and words flow more rapidly after taking alcoholic liquors, people have supposed that this helps brain work. But this activity is untrustworthy. It is a great mistake to think that alcohol in any form will help brain work.[2]

That faculty of the mind that decides what is good sense, what is right, wise, and best, is called the judgment. Alcohol takes the edge off the judgment. A person whose brain is excited with alcohol will laugh and be greatly pleased with what is in reality foolish, silly, and unwise.

Under this misleading excitement, many persons

[1] See note 12, page 237.   [2] See note 13, page 238.

have uttered words and performed deeds that filled
them with shame to recall when the effects of the
alcohol had passed off. Many a life that might otherwise have been one of happy usefulness, has been
permanently disgraced by some act performed under
this first flush, when alcohol had dulled the sense of
right. Many and many a success in life has been lost,
because he who should have been the man of the hour
was unfit for duty from having dulled his brain with
alcohol.

If still more alcohol is taken, those functions which
are under the direct control of the spinal cord become
disturbed. The power over some of the muscles is
lost. The muscles of the lower lip and of the legs are
the first to feel this lack of control. The speech is
thick, and the gait uncertain. Reason is off duty, and
the lower or animal impulses begin to manifest themselves. The control of the judgment and of the will is
lost ; and the emotional, the impulsive, and the purely
instinctive parts of the nature are excited and act without a master. Cruel deeds and crime are the result.

In the last stage of all, when the drinker has become
dead drunk, the paralysis of the nerve centres and of
the brain is carried to its full extent. All the inlets of
the senses are closed, consciousness and sensation are
lost, and control of the voluntary movements is gone.

112. **Effect of Alcohol upon the Will.** — When a
person with determination does what he undertakes in
spite of difficulties, we say he has a strong will. Without such a will, rightly guided, no one can accomplish
much in life.

Remember this as a golden text all the days of your life : —

ALCOHOL INJURES EVERY FACULTY OF THE MIND, AND ESPECIALLY WEAKENS THE WILL.

The judgment of the drinker often points to the fact that alcohol is injuring his health and character, that it is making him careless about doing right, about attending to his business, and about caring for those dependent upon him. Conscience urges him never to take another drop. He solemnly resolves that he never will.

In the hours of temptation that are sure to follow, the drinker needs a strong will with which to say No, and to keep on saying No, very determinedly, to the appetite that asks for more.

But alas! alcohol has not only the power to create this appetite, as we have seen, but also to weaken the will of the drinker, who is struggling to resist its awful craving.

The person who stands before his "first glass," as well as the occasional drinker, should remember that this awful appetite and weakened will are the natural consequences of the use of alcoholic liquors in any form, and that the time when a person could stop drinking if he would, leads on to the time when he would stop drinking if he could.

When the control of the judgment and the will is destroyed by alcohol, cruelty, anger, and other brutal passions are let loose without a master. Thus the drinker becomes an utter slave to his lower nature, and often a terror to those whom he should protect.

The most brutal crimes are often committed while a

person is crazed with strong drink.[1] The craving for ardent spirits becomes well-nigh irresistible. Self-respect, honor, conscience, common decency, — everything is sacrificed to get fresh fuel for the alcoholic fire which is burning up its victim.

The disease known as *delirium tremens*, meaning "a trembling madness," is a terrible example of the profound effect which alcohol may have upon the nervous system. It is marked by muscular tremors, persistent wakefulness, muttering talk, wild delirium, and all the horrors of hideous delusions which the imagination can possibly conceive.

These extreme instances of the breaking-up of the nervous system are found in "homes for the intemperate" and in our insane-asylums, — men and women who have lost every better trace of humanity, hopeless, helpless, doomed to a living death until they cease to breathe.

113. The Inherited Craving for Alcohol. — The craving for alcohol may be inherited by its victim's innocent children, just as we inherit mental and physical vigor or weakness, our features, and even our moral traits. The inherited curse from strong drink has caused many a family to "run out," and leave the children and grandchildren pitiable wrecks of humanity.

There is a marked tendency in nature to transmit all diseased conditions. But of all agents, we must remember that alcohol is the most potent in establishing a heredity that shows itself in the destruction of mind and body.[2] Children often inherit small, weak brains, and a tendency to crime and insanity from the alcoholic habits of their parents.

1 See note 14, page 239.   2 See note 15, page 240.

114. The Use of Tobacco. — The enormous use of tobacco is well known, whether smoked, chewed, or used as snuff. However used, it is a narcotic and a poison. Its injurious effects are due to its "nicotine," which is one of the most rapidly fatal poisons known, rivalling prussic acid in this respect.

It takes about one minute for a single drop of nicotine to kill a full-grown cat, and it has killed a rabbit in three minutes. The application of tobacco to chafed surfaces, and even to the healthy skin, occasions severe and sometimes fatal results. A tea made of tobacco and applied to the skin has caused death in three hours. Soldiers have been known to shirk military duty by making themselves sick with a leaf of tobacco put under the arm or over the stomach.

The injury done by tobacco varies according to the quantity used. Even in moderate use it is hurtful, especially to young persons, and the tobacco habit once acquired is difficult to break. The appetite for it grows with its use. The fact that the habit is foolish, costly, and ill becoming, needs no physiological proof.

Tobacco often produces palpitation of the heart, certain forms of dyspepsia, irritation of the throat and lungs, and a general breaking-up of the nervous system. Sometimes, after long smoking, a feeling of dizziness, with a brief loss of consciousness, is produced. At other times, if walking, there is a sense of falling forward, or as if the feet were sinking into cotton-wool.

Tobacco has the power to injure the brain. Ideas lack clearness of outline. The will-power is weakened, till it is an effort to do the routine duties of every-day life.[1] The tobacco-user is often cross, irritable, and liable to outbursts of passion. The memory is also often impaired : the nicotine deadens the delicate nerve-tissue, and hinders its nutrition. The nerve centres are no longer able to hoard up the necessary amount of vital energy, hence the many and various nervous symptoms due to the use of tobacco.

115. **Effect of Tobacco upon Young People.** — Tobacco in any form has a peculiarly injurious effect upon young people. It seriously impairs muscular growth and mental activity. The profound effect it has upon the nervous system after the first trial of smoking or chewing is well known.

Even after the system gets used to tobacco, young people continue to suffer from nausea, dizziness, headache, muscular trembling, loss of appetite, and general weakness. No boy can continue the practice of smoking or chewing without becoming physically or mentally injured by the time he is twenty-one.

This is the whole story in a nut-shell : No person should learn to smoke, or use tobacco in any way, especially if he wishes to keep strong and vigorous, or is ambitious to succeed in life.

116. **Cigarettes and the Harm they do.** — The use of cigarettes cannot be too severely condemned. These are made of the cheapest materials, which are often adulterated with refuse substances, and even with opium. Cigarettes are so common and so cheap that their use to an injurious extent by thousands of young

[1] See note 16, page 240.

people is becoming a very serious matter. Every few days the newspapers contain an account of the death of some boy caused by the use of cigarettes.

Any honest physician will vouch for the accuracy of the following picture : " A fine healthy boy of from twelve to fifteen years of age, well known for his fine physique, even disposition, and great strength, starts in his career as a cigarette-smoker, and what are the results ? The decay of physical power, emaciation, irritable temper, sallow complexion, drawn and anxious look, unsteadiness of hand, dyspepsia, capricious appetite, aversion to parental and other advice, tendency to seek lower companionship.

" More especially in those predisposed to diseases of the nervous system does this rapid decay make itself apparent, and in varying degrees according to the amount of the indulgence. Physicians daily watch this process with pain and anxiety for those intrusted to their care."

117. **The Use of Tobacco from a Moral Point of View.** — Tobacco has the power, through its effect upon the brain and nerves, to deaden the user's affection for his family and friends as well as his sense of politeness, or propriety as to the rights of others. All have a right to pure air to breathe.

The smoker puffs his tobacco smoke into the faces of people on the street-cars and ferries, in waiting-rooms, hotels, and places of amusement, regardless of the fact that it may be very disagreeable.

The tobacco-chewer, selfishly thinking of no one but himself, defiles the floor, stairs, sidewalks, and even stoves and other objects that come within the range of his disgusting habit.

118. Opium. — Opium is the dried juice of the white poppy. Morphine is a white powder made from opium. A solution of opium in alcohol is called laudanum. Paregoric is a weak form of opium combined with other things.

Various forms of **opium** are generally used in liniments, cough-killers, soothing-sirups, stomach-bitters, cholera-mixtures, and countless other preparations which people are eager to buy, hoping for relief from some real or fancied ailment.

Opium is becoming as great a curse to some of the natives of Asia as alcohol and tobacco are to Europe and America. But its use is gaining ground in these countries as well, and for this reason all should know that it is a dangerous narcotic, with power to create an uncontrollable appetite for more.

A person may begin in the most innocent way to use opium to relieve pain ; little by little the meshes of this fascinating narcotic are woven about him. A person cannot leave off its use without the greatest effort. A craving is created, which no one can realize unless he has once felt the power of this drug. Eaten or smoked habitually, to gratify the craving, it makes a living death for its victim. To quit it is untold misery ; to continue it is certain death.

Opium completely changes its victim. A man once upright and honest will lie, cheat, or commit any crime, to get a dose of the fatal drug. Promises and resolutions to stop its use may be sincerely made, but are no more binding than ropes of sand. The deepest melancholy settles on the opium-eater ; and life, once full of joy and happiness, is indeed a heavy burden.

119. **Practical Points about Opium.** — Opium is often given to infants and children in the form of the so-called soothing-sirups, cough-killers, and cholera-mixtures. However soothing the effect may be; the child is simply drugged, and not cured. The practice of giving any opiates for summer complaints, and other household ways of using opium, should be sparingly and very cautiously resorted to.

Children, as a rule, and many grown-up people too, are very susceptible to the action of opium. Young boys have been made stupid, and their health seriously endangered, by smoking cigarettes that have been drugged with opium.

Above all things, do not give to others, especially to children, any opium mixture that has been prescribed for some one else.

120. **Chloral and other Powerful Drugs.** — Chloral is a powerful drug, capable of producing sleep. Because it is known to induce sleep, especially in those who suffer from excessive mental strain, from anxiety, or other like cause, it has come of late years to be often used without a physician's advice. Like all narcotics, the dose must be steadily increased to get the required effect.

The "chloral habit" is soon formed, and the person becomes a slave to a dangerous drug. Without it the chloral-taker cannot sleep : with it his digestion is

sadly out of order. He suffers from dyspepsia, short-
ness of breath, and palpitation of the heart. The
habit begets carelessness in its use, and the fatal dose
is so uncertain that chloral-takers often die from an
overdose.

The only safe rule is, never to touch so dangerous a
drug unless prescribed by a skilful physician.

Now you must know that the epidemic commonly
known as "la grippe," which recently made such sad
havoc with life and health of people the world over,
brought into use a new group of medicines. They are
only known by their scientific names as "antipyrine,"
"antifebrin," and so on. These powerful drugs have
come of late into extensive household use. Let them
severely alone. Good physicians prescribe them only
with the greatest caution.

CHAPTER XI

THE FIVE GATEWAYS OF KNOWLEDGE

121. **How the Brain learns what takes Place in the Outer World.** — Some nerves, as we have learned, control the action of the muscles; others carry a variety of impressions from every part of the body to the brain. When the brain receives a distinct impression through certain nerves, we become conscious of a **sensation.** Exactly how it occurs is one of the many mysteries of our bodily life.

Most sensations are produced by something outside of us. Thus, if we hear a child cry or a bird sing, we have a sensation of sound; if we put sugar on the tongue, hold a rose to the nose, or prick the skin, certain organs receive the impressions, then faithful nerves carry them to the brain, and we thus become conscious of these different sensations.

There are five "gateways" through which the brain learns what takes place in the outer world; in other words, we have five special senses, — **touch, taste, smell, hearing,** and **sight.**

122. **Touch.** — The simplest of the senses is **touch.** It is given to some extent to the whole body; but it is more delicate in the hands and fingers than elsewhere. When we pass our fingers over an object, we say we

have felt it, and can tell if it is soft or hard, rough or smooth.

If we look carefully at the palm of the hand or at the inner surface of the finger or thumb, we see it is grooved in tiny furrows. At the tips of the fingers these furrows form circles, growing larger and larger. If the finger-tips be smeared with ink, an impression can be made on paper, showing these widening circles. In these furrows are the nerves, which are exquisitely sensitive.

In old times, before the art of writing, and therefore of signing one's name, was common, the old English kings, to sign a document, would ink the end of the thumb and stamp it on the paper : hence the phrase, " my *hand* and seal."

This sense can be cultivated to a marvellous extent. Think what blind people can do ! They read rapidly by running their fingers over slightly raised letters, and recognize their friends by feeling their faces. Watch an expert pianist, and see the skill and the precision with which he handles many keys in a few seconds of time.

123. **Taste.** — The tongue is the principal organ of taste. It has two coverings, — an outer layer, and a deep, sensitive layer. In some diseases this outer layer becomes coated with a whitish or yellowish matter. The deep layer is raised up, like the true skin, into tiny hillocks, or *papillæ*, which are abundantly supplied with delicate nerves, — the nerves of taste.

The tip and back of the tongue are supplied with different nerves. Hence it makes a difference whether we put a substance to be tasted, on the tip or back of the tongue. Thus alum tastes acid on the tip, and has a sweetish taste on the back part of the tongue.

In certain animals these papillæ are very large, and give a roughness to the tongue. We know how rough a cat's tongue is. It is this which enables the cat to strip off the flesh from a bone by simply licking it, while the lion strips the skin from his victim with one stroke of his tongue.

Taste is very much a matter of custom. The Laplanders drink rancid fish-oil with a relish; the Persians used as an appetizer the offensive assafœtida, which

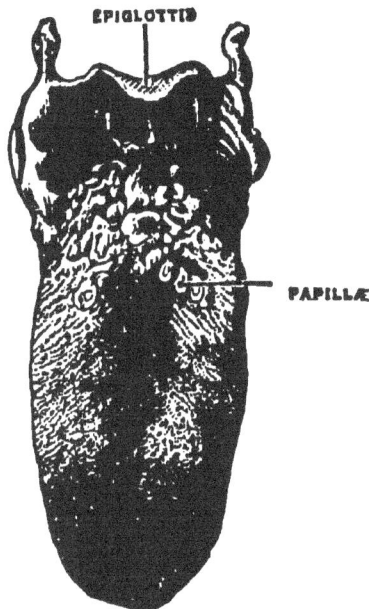

FIG. 47. — Upper Surface of the Tongue, showing the Papillæ.

they called the divine perfume; and the Chinese season their salad with castor-oil. Great acuteness may be gained in the sense of taste. The skill of the "tea-tasters" is something wonderful.

124. Smell. — The seat of the sense of smell is in the cavities of the nose, into which the nostrils open, and which connect behind with the back part of the mouth. The walls of the nasal cavities are lined with a thick, velvety membrane, over which the nerves of smell are distributed.

This membrane is kept continually moist by a fluid

which it secretes. At the beginning of a cold in the head, this membrane becomes dry and swollen, and the

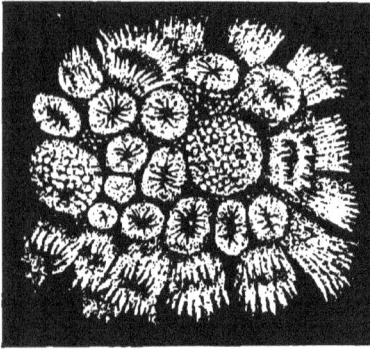

FIG. 48. — How the Papillæ of the Tongue look under the Microscope.

sense of smell is lessened. In the roof of the nasal cavities, the sense of smell is most acute : hence, when we wish to detect a faint odor, we sniff up the air.

The sense of smell varies very much in different individuals ; in some persons it is very dull, while others have a very "sharp nose." In savage races this sense is most acute. We are told that the South-American Indians can by their sense of smell detect the approach of a stranger, even in a dark night, and can also distinguish whether he is white or black.

Many animals are more highly endowed with this sense than man. A dog will smell the footsteps of his master amid those of a hundred other people, and can trace him for miles, although he has been for hours out of sight. Pointers also scent game at a great distance.

The sense of smell is nature's sentinel to guard against taking improper food into the stomach, and impure air into the lungs.

125. Hearing. — Next to sight, **hearing** is the most important of the senses. We could get along without being able to taste ; but without seeing and hearing, life would be almost a blank. Our ears have their delicate structure securely lodged in the " temple " bones.

The *outer ear* is a piece of gristle covered with skin, and curiously moulded for catching sounds.   In animals it is quite movable : hence the timid rabbit and the intelligent horse " prick up their ears " to listen.   The

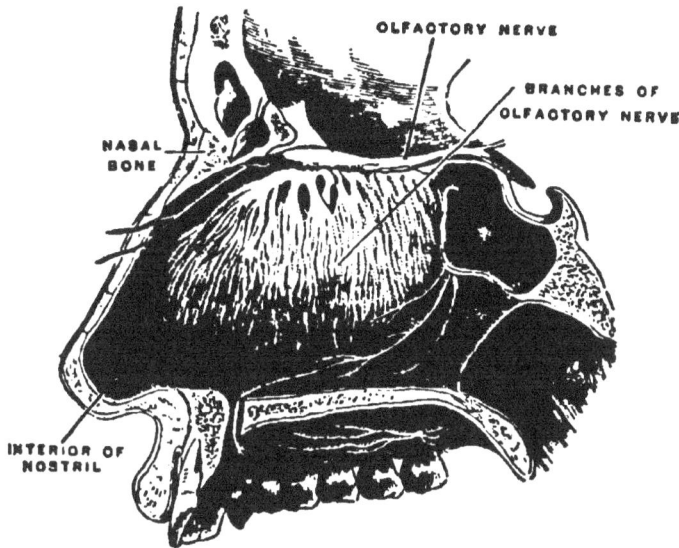

FIG. 49. — Sectional View of the Nose.

tube in the ear is about an inch long, and guides the sound in just as an ear-trumpet does.

At the lower end of this passage we find a delicate membrane stretched across, which serves as a partition between the outer and the middle ear.   It is thin and elastic, hence easily broken by a blow or by pushing anything into the ear.   If once broken or destroyed, deafness results.

The *middle ear* is really the "drum," and in form resembles an ordinary drum.   Three of the tiniest bones in the body stretch across it.   They are so small that you can easily balance them on the tip of your finger. One curious thing is, that they are as large in infancy as they ever will be.

The air reaches the inside of our " ear-drum " through a little tube about an inch long, which leads into it from the throat. It serves to keep the air on both sides of the drum at a constant and even pressure. Hence gunners open their mouths when a heavy cannon is about to be fired, so that the shock may be felt less forcibly. In going up a high mountain or down in a diving-bell, people swallow repeatedly, to save the feeling of discomfort and pain in the ears.

The *inner ear* is one of the most delicate and complex pieces of mechanism in the whole body. It is really a bony case of the tiniest winding chambers and spiral tubes hollowed out in the solid bone. These little passages are lined with a delicate bag of membrane of exactly the same shape as themselves.

The nerve of hearing passes from the brain, through a little hole in the skull to the inner ear, and is spread out on this lining. The impression thus perceived is carried to the brain, where it gives rise to the sensation of hearing.

126. How to take Care of the Ears. — The ear is a very delicate organ. It is often carelessly and ignorantly tampered with. It is often neglected when skilled treatment is urgently needed. The ear-canal should never be rudely or hastily washed out, but the utmost gentleness used in cleansing it.

Children's ears should never be pulled or boxed, for even a slight blow has resulted in deafness. Never use ear-picks, ear-spoons, the end of pencils or penholders, pins, hairpins, toothpicks, and so on, to pick or scratch the ear-canal. It is a foolish, needless, and dangerous practice.

Wads of absorbent cotton may be gently put into the ears to shield them from the cold, or they may be worn

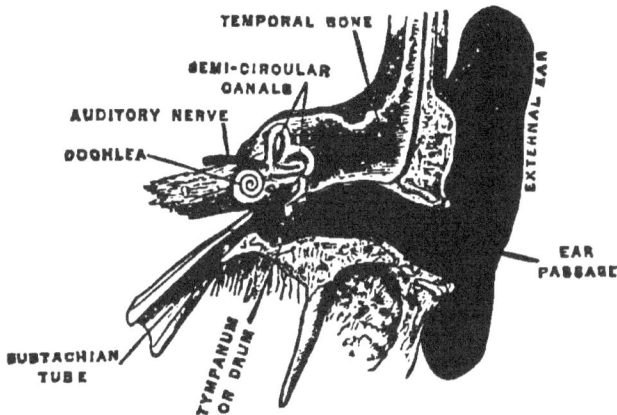

FIG. 50. — Sectional View of the Ear.

in bathing or diving to keep the water out. Diving in deep water, or bathing in the breakers, often injures the ears.

If flies, bugs, ants, and the like crawl into the ears, this may cause some pain and fright, and perhaps lead to vomiting and even convulsions. The ear may then be syringed out with a little warm soapsuds, or drop in a few drops of molasses or sweet oil. Cold water should never be put into the ears, but only tepid water. Do not go to sleep with the head in any position that may expose the ears to a draught of cold or damp air.

127. **Sight.** — Sight, or vision, when we think about it, is a wonderful thing. That we have a means by

which we can learn what is going on in the outside world, miles away from us, is a precious gift.

We watch a huge balloon from the time it leaves the ground till it is a black speck in the air above us. We watch a vessel sailing along on the dim horizon, and the next instant we are reading the fine print of a newspaper. We are able to recognize the form, size, color, and distance of thousands of different objects in nature.

This sense is so woven into the countless acts of our every-day affairs, that we scarcely appreciate this marvellous gift, so essential not only to the simplest matters of comfort, but also to the culture of the mind, and the higher forms of pleasure. Sight is well held to be the highest and most perfect of all the senses.

128. The Eye and its Wonders. — The eye, a most beautiful and ingeniously contrived organ, is the instrument of sight. It is really one of the greatest wonders of nature.

All the seeing parts of the eye are held in an egg-shaped bag lodged in a cavity of the skull. It is well protected by the strong bones of the head. Passing to the brain, through a crevice in the bottom of the cavity, is the *optic nerve*, which gives the power of sight. It spreads itself like a network upon the inner surface of the eyeball, and is then called the retina. It is upon this that the pictures of all objects are thrown. The impression of the pictures is carried to the brain, and causes the sensation of sight.

We must remember that it is not the eye that sees, but the mind behind it ; it is not the ear that hears, but the mind through the ear. This network also takes in the most delicate shades of color ; and by the action of the nerves of both eyes at the same time, we get the idea of the shape of objects, and of their distance from each other.

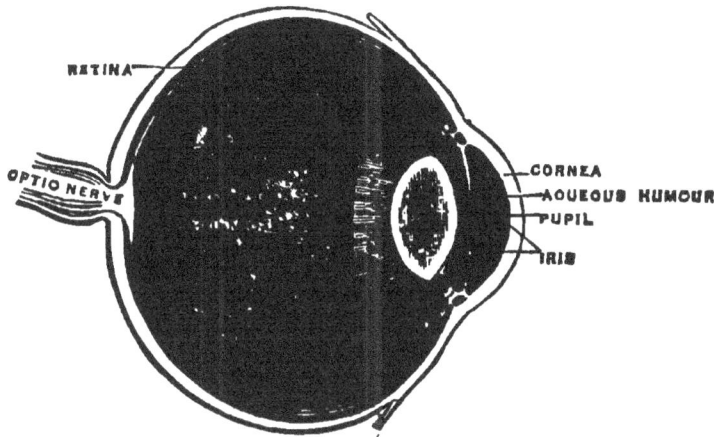

FIG. 51. — Section of Eyeball.

Sometimes the optic nerve is diseased, and total blindness results. The great poet John Milton suffered from this disease, and in his blindness dictated to his daughters the immortal poem, " Paradise Lost."

The eyeball is a bag almost round, thick and dull everywhere but in front, where it has a transparent covering called the *cornea*, meaning a "horn." This is fitted into the eye just as a watch-crystal is fitted into a watch.

Sometimes it bulges out a trifle too much, and an imperfect picture is made on the retina. Such a person is said to be near-sighted. Through this watch-glass the rays of light pass into the ball of the eye. Behind it is a space, called the front chamber of the eye, filled with a watery fluid.

In this chamber hangs a curtain called the *iris*, meaning "rainbow." It has through its centre a hole called the pupil, poetically called "the apple of the eye." This curtain gives the color to the eye.

Behind the pupil is a transparent, jelly-like body, about the size of a French bean, called the *crystalline lens*. It separates the front chamber of the eye from the back chamber. This beautiful lens helps the cornea to bring the pictures to a point, or "focus," on the retina. The back chamber also holds a jelly-like fluid, called the "glassy humor," which allows the iris-curtain to float and move freely.

129. How the Eye is protected. — The eye is like a precious gem placed in a carefully prepared case. The eyelids, by continually winking, protect the eye from insects and from dust. They are fringed with the delicate hairs of the eyelashes, which are so sensitive that the slightest touch gives warning, and the lids close.

By means of little muscles the eye is moved up and down, and rolled sideways. Sometimes these muscles do not act properly, and a person is said to squint or be cross-eyed.

At the upper and outer side of each eye is a little gland which is constantly forming a saltish kind of fluid. Sometimes more of this fluid comes out of the little gland than can be carried away through the nose, and it flows over the eyelids down the cheeks, and is called tears.

Tears are constantly passing over the front of the eye, washing it clean, and keeping it moist; while the eyelid wipes it dry, as it were, by forcing the tears into a little drain-pipe, which carries them off into the nose. Nature, however, kindly oils the edges of the eyelids, to prevent, to some extent, the overflow of tears.

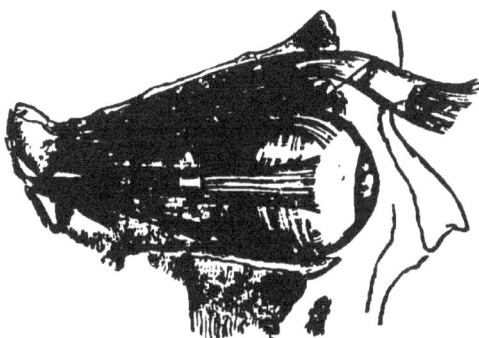

FIG. 52. — Muscles of Eyeball.

130.   **Color-Blindness.** — Color-blindness is the inability to tell certain colors.   It is sometimes produced by sickness, but generally exists at birth.   This defect of sight is quite common.   It is found that four or five out of every hundred people are color-blind.   A person may be color-blind, and not know it until the defect is accidentally revealed.

It is a matter of the utmost practical importance to those employed on railroads, vessels, and other places where colored signals are used.   Some are only partially color-blind, while others are wholly so.   The most common form of color-blindness is that in which one fails to distinguish red.

131. How to take Care of the Eyes. — The eye is an exceedingly delicate and sensitive organ. It is easy to get it out of order, and very tedious to restore it to health. The eyes are often weak after certain sicknesses, especially measles and scarlet-fever. The habit of reading in the cars or a carriage the daily papers, with their blurred and fine print, is a severe strain on the eyes.

It is a dangerous practice to read in bed at night, or while lying down in a darkened room. The small type and poor paper of the many cheap books now so popular, are very frequent causes of weak and diseased eyes.

The direction in which the light comes is an important matter. The worst of all is from in front. The direct light should fall upon the print from above and behind, and from the left side. After reading steadily for some time, we should rest the eyes, even for only a minute, by looking at some distant object.

A person should never read, write, sew, stitch, or otherwise use the eyes, when they tingle or smart, or the sight is dim or blurred; for they are weary, and need rest. Using the eyes at dusk, or by artificial light in the early morning, often leads to serious disorders of vision.

The eyes should never be rubbed or handled roughly, much less when they are irritated by some foreign substance. The sooner such is removed, the better. Rubbing the eye, or pulling the eyelids, only makes a bad matter worse.

Remember this bit of advice: It is not a wise economy to tamper with one's eyes when they are ailing.

132.   Effect of Alcohol and Tobacco on the Special Senses. — Whatever dulls or weakens the nerves, must exert the same effect upon the special senses.

Hence alcohol and tobacco dull the senses, and also provoke changes in the sense-organs themselves.   Thus alcohol often injures the ears by inflaming the throat, and then the tube which leads to the middle ear.

Tobacco is apt to cause an inflamed state of the throat and nose, and hence ear-disease.   Smokers occasionally suffer from a dimmed vision due to a partial paralysis of the optic nerve.   Alcohol is said to cause the same disease.

Tobacco and alcohol often produce an inflammation of the eyes and of the lining of the lids.

Cigarettes are said to be especially hurtful to the lining of the throat, and the eyes.   An atmosphere loaded with tobacco smoke is apt to provoke an inflammation of the throat, nose, and ears.

The power of tobacco to injure the eye is not confined to the user himself.   Careful observers are of the opinion that much of the weak and imperfect vision in the young to-day may be traced to the smoking habits of their fathers.

CHAPTER XII

HELP AT HAND: OR WHAT TO DO IN ACCIDENTS OR ILLNESS

133. Accidents and Emergencies. — Any kind of accident and emergency may happen. When such arise it is necessary to think and to act at a moment's notice.

A friend may cut himself with a scythe or a knife; a child may accidentally swallow some poison; a boy may be taken out of the river apparently drowned; one of our own family may be sick with some contagious disease, or may be nearly suffocated with coal-gas.

All these, and many other things of a like nature, call for a cool head, a steady hand, and some practical knowledge of the best thing to do "till the doctor comes."

Every one should become familiar with a few of the simplest helps in ordinary accidents, emergencies, and in other matters pertaining to every-day health: it is really the practical application of what we have studied in this little book.

134. What to do for a Fainting Person. — A fainting person should be laid flat at once, with the head very low. Give plenty of fresh air; and dash cold water, if necessary, on the head and neck. Loosen all tight clothing.

135. Frostbite. — The ears, toes, nose, and fingers are occasionally frostbitten or frozen. Rub the frozen parts gently with snow or snow-water, in a cold room. The circulation should be restored very slowly. Hot milk with cayenne pepper, and ginger tea, should be freely given as stimulants.

136. Fits, Convulsions. — A sufferer from "fits" should be treated much the same as for fainting. There is foaming at the mouth, the eyes are rolled up, and the tongue or lips are often bitten.

See that the person does not injure himself; crowd a folded handkerchief between the teeth, to prevent biting the lips or tongue. Persons who are subject to such fits should not go into crowded or excited gatherings of any kind.

137. Suffocation. — The chief dangers from poisoning by noxious gases come from the fumes of burning coal in the furnace, stove, or range; from gas blown out by a draught; from the foul air often found in old wells; and from the fumes of charcoal and the foul air of mines.

The first thing to do is to give fresh air. Remove the person to the open air, loosen all tight clothing, dash on cold water, and, if necessary, use artificial respiration, as stated in Section 151.

138. Broken Bones. — Send for a surgeon at once. Loss of power, pain, and swelling are symptoms of a broken bone, that may be easily recognized.

Broken limbs should always be handled with great care and tenderness. If the accident happens in the woods, the limb should be bound with handkerchiefs, suspenders, or strips of clothing, to a piece of board, pasteboard, or bark, padded with moss or grass, which will do well enough for a temporary splint. Always put a broken arm into a sling after the splints are on.

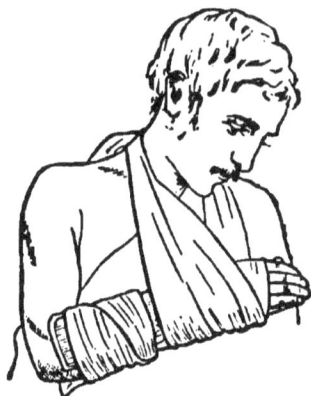

Never move the injured person until the limb is made safe from further injuries by putting it into splints. If you do not need to move the person, keep the limb in a natural, easy position, until the doctor comes.

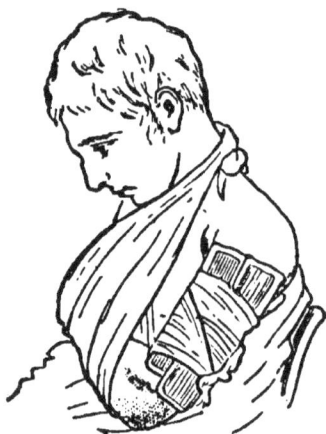

Remember that this treatment for broken bones is only to enable the patient to be moved without further injury. A surgeon is required to set the broken limb.

FIG. 53. — Showing how a temporary splint and a sling may be put on to a broken arm.

Keep the patient warm. Do not give a drop of alcoholic liquor.

139. The Sting of Insects. — If a piece of the sting remains in the wound, extract it with the fingers or with a pair of tweezers. The best application is diluted ammonia-water, after which a cloth moistened with sweet-oil or cosmoline should be placed upon the part.

140. Nosebleed. — Slight nosebleed requires little treatment. Keep the head erect, place a basin under the chin for the blood to run into, and then the patient should take several deep inspirations, filling the chest fully at each breath. In most cases this will soon stop the bleeding. Ice may be applied to the nose.

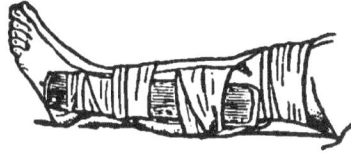

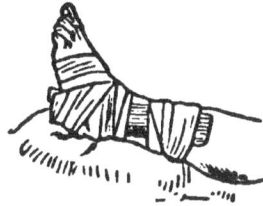

141. Foreign Bodies in the Nose. — Children are apt to push marbles, beans, peas, fruit-stones, buttons, and other small objects, into the nose. Sometimes we

FIG. 54. — Showing how a temporary splint may be put on to a broken leg.

can get the child to help by blowing his nose hard. At other times a sharp blow between the shoulders will cause the substance to fall out. Stop the well nostril, and blow suddenly and forcibly through the mouth.

Call in medical help at once if you do not meet with success, especially if it is a pea or bean, which is apt to swell with the warmth and moisture.

142. Foreign Bodies in the Ear. — The simplest thing to do is to syringe in a little warm water, which will often wash out the substance. If insects crawl into the ear, drop in a little sweet-oil or molasses. If the tip of the ear is pulled up gently, the liquid will flow in more readily.

143. Foreign Bodies in the Throat. — Bits of food and other small objects sometimes get lodged in the throat, and are easily got out by the forefinger or by sharp slaps on the back. If it is a sliver from a toothpick, a match, or a fish-bone, it is no easy matter to remove it ; for it generally sticks into the lining of the passage.

If the object has actually passed into the wind-pipe, and then occur sudden fits of spasmodic coughing, with a dusky hue to the face and fingers, there is great danger of life : surgical help must be called without delay.

If a foreign body, like coins, pencils, keys, fruit-stones, etc., is swallowed, it is not wise to give physic. Give plenty of hard-boiled eggs, cheese, and butter-crackers, so that the substance may be passed off in the natural way, in a bulky stool.

144. **Foreign Bodies in the Eye.** — Cinders, particles of dust, and other small substances, often get into the eye, and cause much pain. Do not rub the eye ; it will only make bad matters worse. Often a copious flow of tears will wash the substance away ; it is sometimes removed with the twisted corner of a handkerchief carefully used.

If it is not removed, or if not found, in this way, the upper lid must be turned back. This requires skilled help.

145. **Sunstroke or Heatstroke.** — The worst cases of " sunstroke" often happen in places where the sun's rays never penetrate. There is sudden loss of consciousness, with deep, labored breathing, an intense, burning heat of the skin, and a marked absence of sweat.

The main thing is to lower the temperature. Strip

off the clothing. Apply to the head chopped ice wrapped in flannel. Rub ice over the chest, and place pieces under the arm-pits and at the sides. If there is no ice, use cloths wet with cold water. The body may be partially stripped, and sprinkled with ice-water from a common watering-pot.

Persons who have once suffered from sunstroke should avoid any risk in the future.

146. Burns or Scalds. — Remove the clothing with the greatest care. Do not pull, but carefully cut and coax, the clothes away from the burnt places. Save the skin unbroken if possible, taking care not to break the blisters.

The secret of treatment is to avoid chafing, and to keep out the air. Baking-soda, used dry or dissolved in water, is a very good household remedy for burns. Another remedy is to soak strips of old linen in a mixture of half linseed-oil and half lime-water.

Spread cosmoline freely with a table-knife on strips of old linen. Apply to the burnt parts and protect them from the air with bandages, lint, or wads of absorbent cotton. A deep or extensive burn should have prompt medical attendance.

147. Bruises, Cut and Torn Wounds. — A bruise is a wound of the soft parts caused by blows. A black eye, and a lip or finger hurt by a base-ball, are familiar examples. Soak the injured part at first in cloths wrung out in cold water. Very hot water is often used to relieve the pain. If the cuts are small, clean the parts, bring the edges together, and stick them with plaster.

When wounds are made with ragged edges, such as

those made by broken glass, splinters, toy pistols, and rusty nails, more skill is called for.

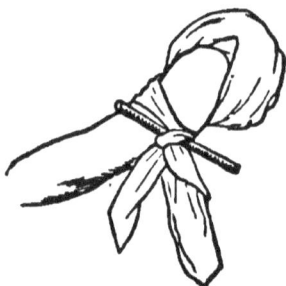

Such wounds, if neglected, often lead to serious results, from blood-poisoning. The services of a doctor are generally necessary.

148. What to do for Bleeding. — It is very important to know the difference between bleeding from an artery and that from a vein.

FIG. 55. — Showing how a handkerchief and a stick may be applied to the arm to stop bleeding.

If an artery bleeds, the blood is of a bright-scarlet color, and spurts in a stream. If a vein bleeds, the blood is of a dark and purple color, and slowly oozes out, or flows in a steady stream.

Bleeding from an artery is a dangerous matter in proportion to the size of the vessel, and life itself may be speedily lost; while bleeding from a vein is rarely a serious injury, and generally stops of itself, aided, if need be, by pressure.

When an artery is bleeding, always remember to *make deep pressure between the wound and the heart.* Send at once for the doctor.

Meanwhile there is something to do. Keep cool, and do not be afraid to act at once. A firm grip in the right place with the fingers will do, until a twisted handkerchief, stout cord, shoestring, or suspender is ready to take its place.

If the artery is of some size, make a knot in whatever is used, and bring the pressure of the knot to bear over the artery. If the flow of blood does not stop, change the pressure until the right spot is found. Strips of an old handkerchief, a bunch of moss, underclothing, or cotton-wadding, might be stuffed into the wound, keeping up the pressure all the time ; or seize a handful of dry earth, and crowd it down into the bleeding wound with a firm pressure.

Let me tell you of the principal places to apply pressure when arteries are injured and bleeding.

If in the *finger*, grasp it with the thumb and forefinger, and pinch it firmly on each side ; if in the *hand* press with the thumb just above, and in front of, the wrist.

For injuries *below the elbow*, grasp the upper part of the arm with the hands, and squeeze hard.

For the *upper arm*, press with the fingers against the inner edge of the biceps muscle.

FIG. 56. — Showing how a bandage may be used to stop bleeding from an artery in the arm.

For the *foot* or *leg*, press as before in the hollow behind the knee, just above the calf of the leg.

149. Apparent Drowning. — Remove all tight clothing from the neck, chest, and waist. Sweep the fore-

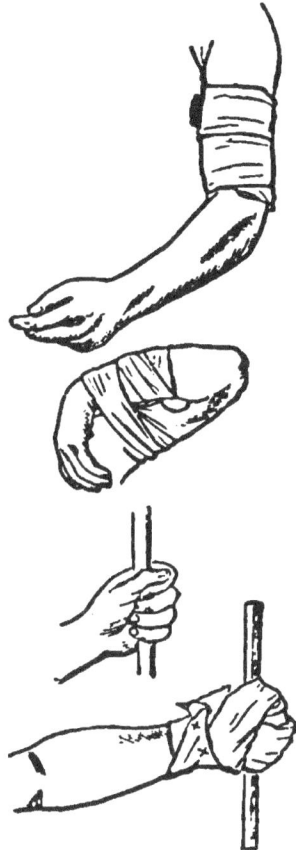

finger, covered with a handkerchief or towel, round through the mouth, to free it from froth and mucus.

Turn the body on the face, raising it a little with the hand under the hips, to allow any water to run out from the air-passages. Take only a moment for this.

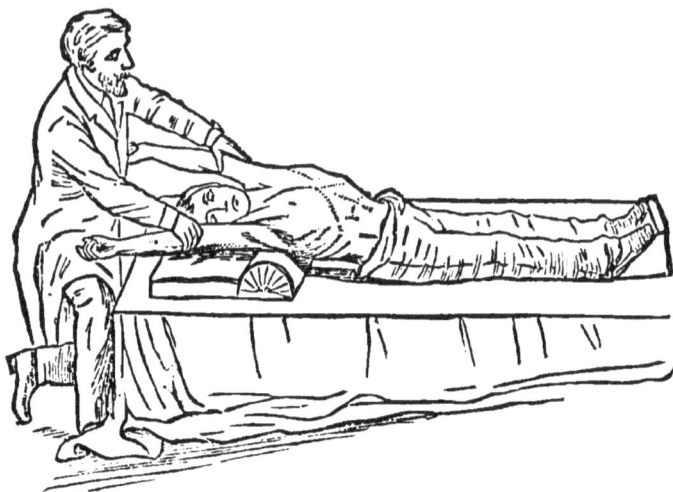

FIG. 57. — The process of artificial respiration : first step.

Lay the person flat upon the back, with a folded coat or pad of any kind, to keep the shoulders raised a little. Remove all the wet, clinging clothing that is convenient.

If in a room or sheltered place, strip the body, and wrap it in blankets, overcoats, etc. Use bottles of hot water, if at hand, hot flat-irons, or hot sand, round the limbs and feet.

The main thing to do is to keep up artificial respiration until the natural breathing comes, or till all hope is lost.

This is the simplest way to do it : The person is

laid on the back. Let some one kneel behind the head. Grasp both arms near the elbows, and sweep them upward above the head until they nearly touch. Make a firm pull for a moment. This tends to fill the lungs with air by drawing the ribs up, and making the chest cavity larger.

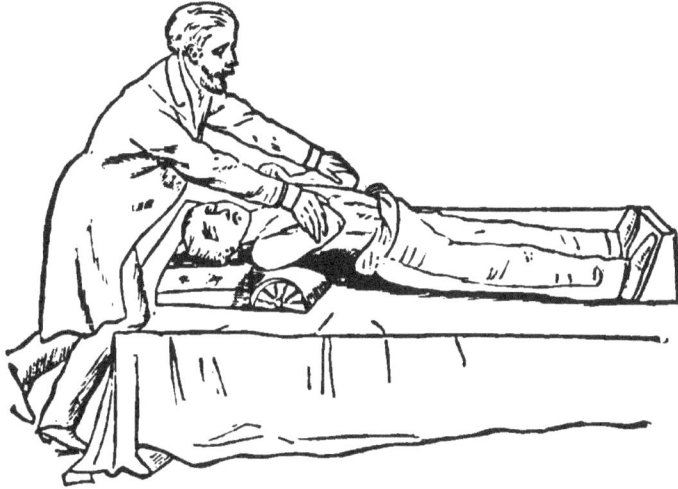

FIG. 58. — The process of artificial respiration : second step.

Now return the arms to the sides of the body until they press hard against the ribs. This tends to force out the air.

This makes, artificially, a complete act of respiration. Repeat this act about fifteen times every minute. All this may be kept up for several hours.

When a person can breathe, even a little, he can swallow. Give then hot, strong coffee every few minutes, a teaspoonful at a time, or a little ammonia and water. Meanwhile do not fail to keep up artificial warmth.

Do not move a person who is just beginning to breathe again from one place to another, except when forced to do so from cold or some pressing necessity.

HINTS AND HELPS FOR EVERY-DAY HEALTH

150. Proper Care of the Bowels. — Irregularity in eating, too much finely bolted flour and not enough fruit and vegetables, rich pastry, negligence in attending to a regular evacuation of the bowels, lead to the very common and distressing trouble known as **constipation.** As we grow older, this trouble generally grows worse.

We should pay strict attention to the proper action of the bowels. The formation of a *regular habit* is of the utmost importance. The bowels can be trained to act at a certain time every day. Eat plenty of coarse food, such as oatmeal, corn-bread, vegetables, stewed prunes, dates, figs, etc. Drink a glass of water just after getting out of bed in the morning.

If these things do no good, consult a physician before unknown medicines are used in a hap-hazard sort of way.

151. The Habit of taking Unknown Medicines. — The habit of taking medicines, especially of an unknown character, is alarmingly common. If we have an ache or pain about us, a friend advises this or that medicine because "it did him good," or we are foolish enough to spend our money for some advertised nostrum claiming to have wonderful virtues.

All people, especially sensible young persons, should have respect enough for their health to let all unknown medicines alone. Rest assured, if the skilful physician cannot help us, medicines made by some "benefactor of mankind," simply to sell, will do us little good.

152. Hints for the Sick-room. — The sick-room should be the lightest and most pleasant room in the house. Take away all extra carpets, upholstered furniture, heavy curtains, etc. : they absorb the impurities, and help keep the room foul. A clean floor, with a few rugs to deaden the footsteps, is much better than a woollen carpet.

Let the room be open to the sunlight and the fresh air. Guard the patient from the noise of passing steam and horse cars, heavy teams, and playing children. With a little pains any sick-room may be supplied with pure air.

Do not let the disagreeable odors due to cooking, especially frying fish or pork, cooking cabbage, etc., reach the sick-room. Do not allow a kerosene light, with its flame turned down, to burn through the night.

Keep a sick-room neat and trim. Remove at once all offensive matters. Never allow such to remain in the room. In many diseases, especially scarlet-fever, diphtheria, consumption, etc., use pieces of old linen instead of handkerchiefs, and burn them as soon as used. Carelessness or ignorance in this matter often spreads contagious disease.

Change the clothes of the bed and of the patient quite often. Do not let such clothing be put away in a closet with other clothing. Put it to soak at once in boiling water, with some disinfectant like Platt's chlorides. Do not have food left in the room.

Do not make a great show of bottles of medicines, spoons, glasses, etc., carefully spread out on the bureau or table. Keep all such things in an adjoining room. To a patient not used to sickness, a great show of drugs and sick apparatus is discouraging. Some simple thing like an orange, a few favorite flowers, and one or two playthings, may take their place.   ·

Never get behind the door, in a corner, or in an adjoining room, and *whisper*. Whatever must be said, say it openly and aloud. Answer a sick person's questions plainly and squarely. Nothing is gained by trying to avoid a straightforward reply.

If a doctor is employed, carry out his orders to the very letter.

153. Sicknesses that spread. — We have learned in a preceding chapter (chap. viii.) that the air may be poisoned by the products of respiration, and by other waste matters thrown off from *healthy* human bodies.

The air may be poisoned also by the products of respiration and bodily discharges of *diseased* persons. Thus, in certain diseases, called *contagious*, there are thrown off in some way from the persons of the sick, organic matters, which tend to reproduce themselves in the bodies of other persons.

Small-pox and scarlet-fever are examples of severe and contagious diseases ; while whooping-cough, measles, and mumps are contagious, but less harmful.

Again : the air may be poisoned with the foul gases

arising from the contents of cesspools, water-closets, sewers, and other sources.

The living particles, or "germs," of such diseases as typhoid-fever and dysentery, are believed to be contained or developed in the discharges both from the stomach and bowels of persons suffering from these diseases. Diphtheria and typhoid-fever are believed to be due oftentimes to the foul contents of cesspools and sewers.

Finally, the air may be poisoned by the decay of organic matters in the ground, and drawn into the house in various ways. Thus there seems to be a connection between typhoid-fever and bad drainage.

154. Disinfection. — With our present knowledge, it is not possible to get rid of the germs of disease after they are once lodged in the body. We are able, however, to a certain extent, to destroy them after they leave the body in the discharges of diseased persons.

This destruction of the poisons of infectious and contagious diseases is called *disinfection*, and the means used are called **disinfectants.** We must remember that disinfection cannot make up for the want of cleanliness or of ventilation.

Practical directions for the use of disinfectants are given in the more advanced text-books.

155. Poisons in General. — Poisons of various kinds are often used in the trades, and kept about the house and premises as medicines, as disinfectants, for killing insects and animals, and for many other purposes.

People are often careless about them, and leave them in the cupboard, or on a shelf about the shed or stable, wrapped in a piece of paper, or in some unlabelled bottle. Children either mistake them, or are urged by some playmate to swallow them.

The many accidents due to drinking carbolic acid by mistake are a familiar example of how stupid or careless people may be.

Poisons should always be carefully labelled, and the word " POISON " plainly printed in large letters across the label.

Fasten the cork firmly to the bottle by wire, twisted into a knot at the top. This would certainly prevent a person from mistaking carbolic acid, ammonia, oxalic acid, etc., in the dark, for medicine.

Poisons should never be kept in the same place with medicines or other bottled preparations used in the household. Put them in some secure place, and under lock and key.

Here is a golden rule : Never use the contents of any package or bottle unless you know exactly what it is. Do not guess at it, or take any chances ; but destroy it at once.

Poisons may be taken when medical help, especially in the country, cannot be had at short notice. They do their work rapidly. Something must be done, and that at once and in earnest.

The stomach must be emptied as speedily as possible. Make a quart of warm soapsuds. Force the sufferer to gulp it down, a cupful at a time. Run the finger or a feather "down the throat," and hasten the vomiting.

A good emetic is made by putting a heaping tablespoonful of ground mustard into a pint of water. Drink a cupful every ten minutes until vomiting is produced. Stir up a handful of powdered alum in a cupful of molasses, and swallow this, a tablespoonful every ten minutes.

Vomiting will do no harm, and the poison may destroy life in a few minutes.

The young student is referred to more advanced text-books than this, for the use of antidotes for particular poisons.

CHAPTER XIII

PRACTICAL EXPERIMENTS

156. Value of Experiments. — To get a proper understanding of the elementary principles of physiology, it is not enough simply to study the text. The same general principles hold as in any other branch of scientific study. A show of suitable specimens and a series of **practical experiments** should supplement the intelligent study of the text proper.

Whatever we see with our eyes, feel with our fingers, and do with our hands, in the matter of experiment and illustration, however simple and homely, is of far more worth than merely studying the printed page. It is more like hard work, to be sure ; but laziness is a poor excuse in this or in any other branch of science.

It is plain that any series of experiments arranged for use in our common schools must be somewhat crude. We must take many things for granted. The observation and experience of medical men, and the experiments of the physiologist in his laboratory, must be relied upon for important data not otherwise easily obtained by young students.

Because we cannot make our experiments with that accuracy and detail as in other branches of science, it by no means follows that we cannot use experiments in elementary instruction in the lower grade of schools. The simplest experiments become, in the hands of the enthusiastic and skilful teacher, of the greatest value and interest. Pupils soon gain a far better knowledge and keep up a livelier interest in the subject if, as we have just said, they see with their own eyes, and handle with their own hands, that which serves to illustrate the subject.

This method of instruction rivets the attention, and keeps alive the interest, of the young pupil ; in fact, it is the true method of cultivating a scientific habit of study. Hence the following experiments, however simple and rude the apparatus, may become helps towards gaining a more thorough knowledge of this important branch of scientific study.

157. Hints and Helps. — If we had our choice in the matter, we should depend, for this part of our study, upon four sets of illustrations, —

(1) The Skeleton and Manikin.

(2) Experiments on the Person.

(3) Charts, Diagrams, and Blackboard Exercises.

(4) A systematic series of simple Experiments performed by the teacher and the pupils.

By all means secure a **skeleton** and **manikin,** by loan or purchase, if possible. It is better to have some of the separate bones than none at all.

We have suggested many ways in which our own person, or that of a friend, may be utilized for the purpose of experiment and observation. The success of this part of the work will depend upon our skill, tact, and common-sense. How much time and effort it is best to devote to this part of the study, depends upon the age and capabilities of the class. Nothing can take its place in getting an accurate and thorough idea of the more essential and practical points of anatomy.

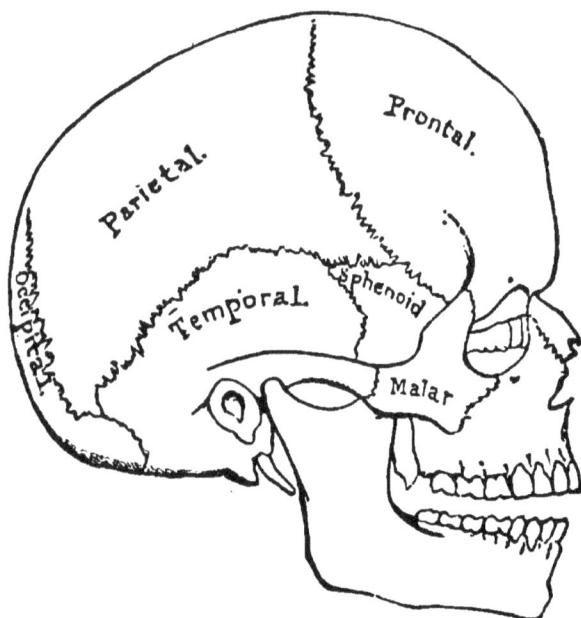

FIG. 59. — BLACKBOARD SKETCH. Right side of the Skull.

The pupil should be trained to make and to copy sketches and diagrams in his note-book, and repeat them at stated intervals on the blackboard. Such sketches may be somewhat rude, and there will be a great contrast in the work of different pupils ; but this is of little account.

The teacher is advised to make for himself a series of diagrams, on a suitable scale for the blackboard, on sheets of manila paper, and have them bound, and hung up for easy reference in the schoolroom, somewhat in the same way that reading charts are now made. These sketches may be used to illustrate the text, and then copied by the pupil in his note-book or on the blackboard.

In addition to this, a set of **physiological charts** is very desirable, and should be secured if possible.

By all means, depend upon a systematic series of rude, homely **experiments.** Most of the experiments in the succeeding pages are simply suggestive. Do not merely copy, but exercise your wits and ingenuity to make others equally good. Most of these experiments can be done with inexpensive and simple apparatus, which can be picked up about the house, the market, and the drug-store.

It is not enough for the pupil to see the teacher make the experiments. Each member of the class should be encouraged to make the experiments.

When specimens of bones, joints, dissections, etc., are carried into the schoolroom, the utmost pains must be taken to keep everything neat and clean. Use large plates, platters, saucers, tissue-paper, with plenty of pins, needles, clean towels, and napkins. Cover every part except what it is necessary to show.

Keep everything covered until the proper time comes. Every little detail must be arranged before the recitation begins. If the fingers get soiled, remove all traces at once. Strict attention to all these little matters may make the difference between success and failure in making these practical experiments.

EXPERIMENTS ON THE BONES

[Chapter II. page 11.]

EXPERIMENT 1. *To show the Gross Structure of Bone.* — Saw lengthwise in two a beef bone. Save one-half. Boil, scrape, and carefully clean the other half. Note in the boiled half the compact and spongy parts, shaft, etc. Note on the other half, the pinkish-white look of the bone, the marrow and its tiny specks of blood, etc., — in other words, the difference between the fresh (live) bone, and an old, dry one (dead) easily found for the purpose.

2. *To show the Animal Part of Bone.* — Get a chicken's leg from the kitchen and put it to soak into a mixture of four tablespoonfuls of muriatic acid to one pint of water. A wide-

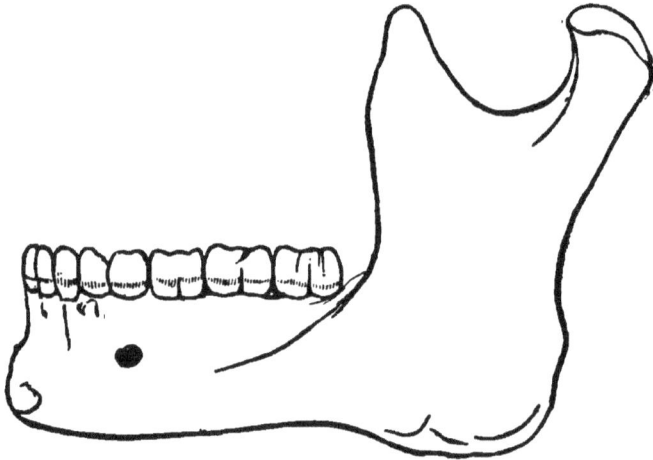

FIG. 60. — BLACKBOARD SKETCH. Side view of the Lower Jaw.

mouthed bottle is the best thing to hold it; next, an earthen bowl. Soak from five days to a week.

It can now be bent, twisted, and even tied into a knot, showing that the earthy matter has been dissolved.

3. *To show the Earthy, or Mineral, Part of Bone.* — Take the second half of the bone from Experiment 1 and roast it on a bright, hot, coal fire for three hours. The animal matter has now been burned out. The earthy part, a white, brittle mass, is now seen, showing every outline of the bone.

Study of the Skeleton. — We shall now proceed to study the skeleton in two ways, — first, upon the mounted skeleton made for such use ; second, by the examination of the skeleton or bones of our own person, or that of a friend. Whether a skeleton or a chart is used, this drill on the living body is of the greatest importance. Let a boy stand before the class ; and, as the teacher points out on him the various bones and bony landmarks of the body, each one of the class should stand, and do the same on his own person.

Do it all with neatness, tact, and a due regard for the feelings of all concerned. Drill thoroughly until all become perfectly familiar with the location of the most important and accessible bones and landmarks of the body.

4. *The Skeleton. — Its Study as a Whole.* — Point out head, trunk, and limbs ; long, short, flat, and round bones. Note how some bones protect certain parts, how others are built for use, beauty, and protection. Do the same on the person, *so far as it is convenient.* Use the chart or skeleton for the same purpose.

5. *Parts of the Skeleton. — The Head.* — Drill on the skeleton for the bones of the head ; the same on the person. Use the chart.

6. Show how the bones of the skull are jointed ; the sutures ; the plates of bones ; the rough surfaces for the attachment of muscles ; holes and notches for arteries and nerves. If nothing better can be had, get a part or the whole of some animal's skull from the market or even the fields.

7. *The Trunk.* — Note the various bones as before. Trace and count each rib and vertebra.

8. *The Upper Limbs.* — The upper arm, forearm, hand. Experiment exactly the same as before. Every part can be carefully traced on the person.

9. *The Lower Limbs.* — Thigh, lower leg, foot. Experiment as before.

10. *Repair of the Bones.* — Ask some pupil who has broken his arm or collar-bone some time previously to show how well the broken parts have united.

11. *Joints.* — Get a part of a calf's or sheep's leg at the market containing the joint. Open the joint carefully.

Note the sticky joint-oil; the synovial fluid; the glistening surfaces of the ends of the bones; the gristle; cartilages; places where tendons, ligaments, and muscles are fastened.

12. *To show the Various Kinds of Joints.* — Illustrate on the person the fixed and movable joints; ball and socket; hinge; pivot joints. Try the principal joints of the body, and see just how much and what motion they have.

13. *The Ligaments.* — In cutting open the joints, note the tough, firm, and gristly bands, which help hold the bones together. These are the ligaments. Try to tear or wrench them off from the bone, to see how firm and tough they are.

14. *Bony Landmarks of the Body.* — Go over the skeleton or person, and locate with the fingers certain important "bony landmarks," as the angle of the lower jaw; elbow-end of the ulna; wrist-end of the radius; highest point of scapula; lower end of breast-bone; upper end of tibia; lower end of fibula, etc.

Other landmarks will suggest themselves. This will make an excellent review-exercise.

EXPERIMENTS WITH THE MUSCLES

[CHAPTER III. PAGE 31.]

EXPERIMENT 15. *To show the Gross Structure of Muscles.* — Get about half a pound of lean corned beef, a strip with the fibres running all one way. Have it thoroughly boiled. Let it cool, and press it with the weight of several flat-irons. Put it on a firm board or table, and pick it in pieces with two darning-needles.

Note the connective tissue, the larger muscular fibres. Pick with the needles until the fibres are too small to manage.

16. *To show how Muscles look.* — Get the lower part of a sheep's leg at the market, with the foot or hoof still on; dissect with a sharp knife one or more muscles, leaving the insertion. Even if it is roughly done, it is no matter.

17. Use your own biceps and triceps muscles to show how muscles contract and relax, how they oppose each other in action. Repeat the same with other muscles, as the flexors and extensors of the fingers and toes, of the leg, etc.

18. *To show the Structure and Action of Tendons.* — Take some of the material from the previous dissection, and examine the tendons. Get the leg of a fowl at the market, to show the tendons which make the toes bend.

19. Make a study of the tendons on your own person. Grasp the powerful tendons of the hip-muscles under the knee; of the lower leg; near the ankle; of the forearm at the wrist.

20. *To locate some Important Muscles.* — Locate and describe them on the chart. Do the same, as far as it is possible and convenient, on the person. Clutch tightly such muscles as the biceps, deltoid, great pectoral, muscles of the calf of the leg, etc.

21. *Muscular Landmarks.* — Use the chart, skeleton, and person, to locate the most important muscular landmarks, as the origin and insertion of the biceps ; tendon of Achilles ; annular ligament ; edges of the great pectoral and biceps ; flexor cords of the forefinger, etc. This may be made an admirable drill-exercise.

EXPERIMENTS ON FOOD AND DRINK

[CHAPTER IV. PAGE 46.]

A series of most useful experiments may be made on the subject of food and drink. The common articles of diet greet us on every hand. It should be our object to under-stand the *principles* which underlie the matter of daily food. We should become familiar with the principal substances contained in the three great classes of foods.

We can do this by exhibiting specimens, and by experiment. Specimens of the various cereals, starches, sugars, oil, etc., should be shown, which should have been carefully collected and kept for class-use in small radish or pickle bottles. Each specimen should be neatly labelled with its exact name. Many interesting facts can be brought out about the practical use of these substances as foods, when we are able to touch, taste, smell, and see the substances themselves.

22. *To show Albumen.* — The albumens are all rich in one or more of the following organic substances : *albumen, casein, fibrine, gelatine, gluten,* and *legumen.* Boil an egg hard. The white is *albumen* hardened by heat.

23. *To show Casein.* — Pour some liquid rennet, or vinegar, into some milk. A whitish substance (the curd) separates from it. This is *casein,* the chief constituent of cheese.

24. *To show Fibrine.* — Take a piece of lean meat, and

wash it thoroughly in water, squeezing and pressing it well in a lemon-squeezer. A whitish, stringy mass is obtained, which is the *fibrine*. The albumen is dissolved in the water. Boil the water after the meat has been washed. The heat coagulates the albumen.

25. *To show Gelatine.* — Boil a bone a long time. Most of the animal matter will be dissolved. This is *gelatine*.

26. *To show Gluten.* — Put a handful of flour into a muslin bag, and squeeze it well in a basin of water. The water becomes milky; while a sticky, yellowish-white substance remains in the bag. This sticky substance is *gluten*.

27. *To show Legumen.* — Boil a few peas or beans in the pod, until they become a sticky, pulpy mass. This is called *legumen*, and resembles the white of an egg and the gluten of flour.

28. *To show the Starches.* — Specimens of the more common kinds of foods rich in starch, as potato, rice, sago, arrowroot, tapioca, corn-flour, etc., may be used for illustration. The presence of starch is easily proved.

Boil a small quantity of flour, rice, bread, potato, or arrowroot in a little water in a test-tube. Add a drop or two of the tincture of iodine, and the mixture will turn blue.

29. *To show the Sugars.* — *Cane sugar* is familiar as cooking and table sugar. Get some raisins and pick out a handful of the little white grains. This is *grape sugar*. Get a cent's worth of *milk sugar* at the drug store.

30. *To show the Various Kinds of Fats and Oils.* — Show specimens of fats that are solid at ordinary temperatures, such as *beef-suet, mutton-suet, lard,* and *butter.* Liquid fats are commonly called *oils.* The two principal kinds used as food are *olive-oil* and *cod-liver oil.* Get specimens of each at the store.

31. *Simple Experiments to show that Milk is a Model Food.* — Milk is rightly called a compound food, since it is composed

at least five kinds of food-substances. Take some milk "fresh from the cow," and place it in a tall, narrow glass vessel, and allow it to stand for several hours. A quantity of *cream* rises to the top. Cream is the milk-fat. It is simply made up of tiny bags of fat, each of which has a covering of curd. By churning the cream about a short time, the covering is broken, and the little lumps of fat unite to form the yellow solid called *butter*. Now skim off the cream : what remains is called *skim-milk*. Add a teaspoonful of weak vinegar, acid, or liquid rennet, to the skim-milk. Solid whitish lumps of *curd* will be seen separating from a watery fluid called *whey*. We have now divided the milk into three parts, cream, curd, and whey. Cream is the fat; curd is the casein, or nitrogenous part, which, when pressed and dried, is called *cheese;* and whey is *milk-sugar* and *mineral matter* dissolved in *water*.

These simple experiments show that milk contains flesh-forming, bone-making, and heat-giving materials. Remember also, that it contains these in the right proportions, especially for children.

32. *To show Water, the Minerals, and Appetizers.* — *Water* is too familiar a food for experiment.

The mineral matter left from Experiment 3 shows the various kinds of *lime* and *potash*. An egg-shell is a familiar example of *carbonate of lime*. Various kinds of *salt* (forms of soda) can be got from any grocer. The white of an egg contains a little *sulphur*. Leave a silver spoon in it for a short time and the sulphur will blacken it.

Specimens of the most common appetizers should be shown as vinegar, pepper, mustard, ginger, cloves, nutmegs, cinnamon, allspice. etc. ; also samples of substances from which the common beverages are made, such as tea, coffee, cocoa, and chocolate.

EXPERIMENTS WITH ALCOHOL

EXPERIMENT 33. *Alcohol, and how it looks.* — Get at the drug-store a four-ounce white-glass bottle, and let the druggist fill it for you with the best alcohol. Have it tightly corked, and properly marked with a label gummed on the bottom of the bottle.

To remember: Alcohol is a thin, colorless liquid, which looks like water.

34. *To show how Alcohol burns.* — Turn a little alcohol into an old-fashioned fluid lamp. Light it, and note the character of the light and the heat. Put a white saucer or plate closely down on the flame for a few minutes.

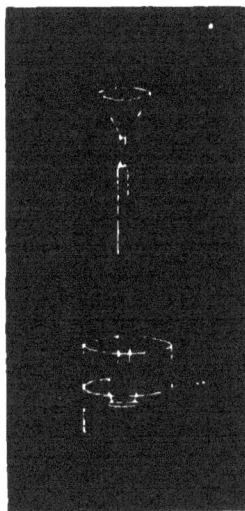

Note that the alcohol burns without soot, giving little light but great heat.

SUGGESTION. — If a fluid lamp is not easily obtained, use a small kerosene lamp without the chimney. A lamp good enough for simple experiments can be made out of a common mucilage bottle, using the hollow handle of the metallic brush for the wick. A piece of a bean-blower run through the cork of an empty horse-radish bottle, using a rolled piece of kerosene-wick for the wick, will also provide the necessary apparatus for an alcohol lamp.

FIG. 61.

35. *To show that Alcohol and Water unite readily, with a Slight Decrease of Volume.* — Use a test-tube which will contain one fluid ounce (eight teaspoonfuls). Drop in thirty drops each of alcohol and water. Gum a strip of white paper four inches long and one-fourth of an inch wide to the

side of the test-tube, bringing the lower end on a level with
the sixty drops of fluid in the tube.   Have the strip of paper
marked off into inches and one-eighths of an inch.

Drop water carefully into the tube until exactly two inches
have been added, as shown on the graduated paper; then drop
in alcohol until exactly two inches more have been added.
Shake the tube carefully, taking care not to spill any of the
fluid.

Note that the alcohol and water unite with a slight decrease
of volume.

36.   *To show the Great Attraction of Alcohol for Water.* —
Tie tightly some thin membrane (like the coverings of the
sausages sold in the markets) across the mouth of a bulb test-
tube.   Place the test-tube (bulb downward) in a goblet or
beaker.   Fill the bulb with alcohol, and pour pure water into
the goblet or beaker (Fig. 67).

The alcohol will soon rise in the tube, thus proving that
alcohol has such a liking for water that it has caused the
water to filter through the membrane.

37.   *To show the Origin of Alcohol in Fermented Liquors.*
— Take a common glass fruit-jar which will hold one pint.
Fill the jar one-half full of water, and add molasses until it
is of a deep-brown color.   Add a teaspoonful of yeast or
one-half of a yeast-cake.   Cover so as to admit some air, and
keep at a temperature of 70° F. for a day or two.

Note the result: The mixture has the odor of alcohol.
What has happened?   Why, the yeast (called a " ferment ")
has changed the sugar of the molasses to alcohol.   The process of changing is called " fermentation."

38.   Use the fruit-jar, as before.   Fill it one-half full of
sweet cider, or squeeze out the juice of a few sweet apples
with a lemon-sqeezer.   Allow the liquid to stand exposed
to warm air for a few days.

Note that the liquid has the peculiar odor of alcohol. This liquid is commonly known as cider. Very minute ferments have changed the sugar of the sweet apple-juice to alcohol. If the liquid is left exposed to the air, it will, after a time, change to vinegar, known by its sour, acid taste.

39. Press out the juice of a few ripe grapes, strain off the skins, and continue as explained in the preceding experiment.

40. Take two wide-mouthed bottles holding one pint each. Be able to connect the two bottles *A* and *B*, as shown in Fig. 62. Let a glass tube run from bottle *B*, and empty into a glass jar (*C*). Use a little putty or sealing-wax to stop any leaks made by the tubing running through the corks.

Fill the bottle *A* about one-half full of molasses. Add one yeast-cake which has been dissolved in water. Fill the bottle with water, and shake vigorously. Fill the bottle *B* nearly full of water.

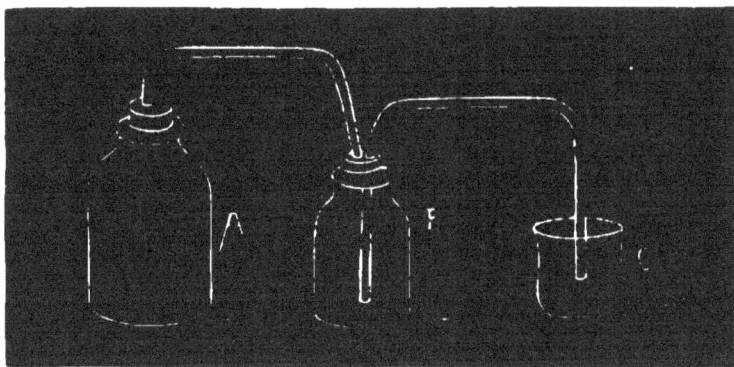

Fig. 62.

Keep the apparatus in a warm room for two or more days; an even temperature of 75° to 80° F. will do.

The pupil will note that the fluid in the bottle *A* soon begins to "work," and that a substance called the lees settles to the bottom of the bottle. The water in bottle *B* will pass up the tube and over into the glass jar *C*. Note also that there is a change in the smell of the liquid. By this change a gas has been formed which has forced the water in *B* over into the glass jar. This change is called fermentation.

41. *To show the Presence of Alcohol in Distilled Liquors.* — Heat hard cider or sherry wine in a large-sized test-tube over an alcohol lamp. Run a piece of glass tube, bent at right

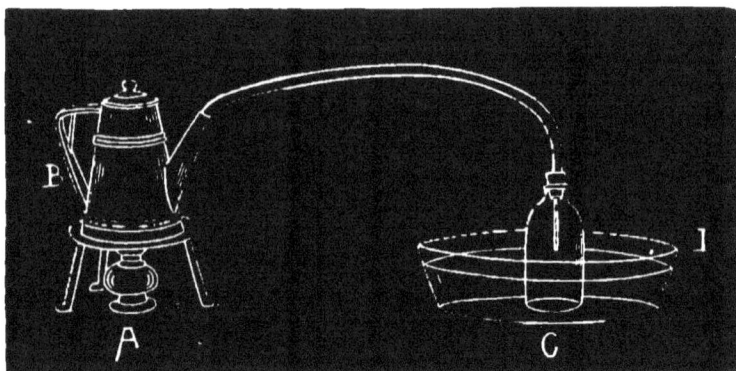

Fig. 63.

angles, through a cork which fits the test-tube; let the other end of the tube be fitted into the cork of a wide-mouthed bottle which is set into a basin of cold water to condense the steam.

The resulting liquid has a marked odor and taste. It is stronger than the fermented liquid. This process is called "distillation," and the resulting liquid, " distilled liquor."

42. Pour one-half of a pint of hard cider into a common tin coffee-pot. Fasten a piece of rubber tubing to the spout. Have the other end of the tubing run into a wide-mouthed bottle sunk into a basin of cold water. Cloths wrung out in ice-water may be wrapped round the bottle. Heat the

cider in the coffee-pot by an alcohol lamp, placed as shown in Fig. 63. Do not allow the cider to boil.

Note that the color and odor of the resulting liquor differ from the color and odor of the hard cider. A stronger liquor has been produced by this process. This process is called distillation. The stronger liquor has been separated from the water. It may be necessary to re-distil the resulting liquor several times before a liquor is found pure enough to burn.

43. *To show the Effect of Alcohol on Albumen.* — Place in an empty quinine or horse-radish bottle the white of an egg. Pour in some strong alcohol. Stir with a spoon or glass rod.

Note that the alcohol hardens, or coagulates, the albumen; in other words, the alcohol has such a liking for the water of the albumen, that it withdraws it, leaving it hard.

44. Repeat the same experiment, using dilute alcohol (one-half alcohol and one-half water).

45. Place in the same kind of a bottle as before a small strip of raw beefsteak. Add strong alcohol, and let mixture be set aside for a few days.

Note that the meat seems hard. The alcohol has coagulated the albumen of the meat. The alcohol withdraws the water of the fresh, elastic, muscular tissue, leaving it tough and hard.

46. Squeeze a piece of fresh beef in a lemon-squeezer over a wide-mouthed bottle. Pour in a little water; stir it until well colored with blood. Add strong alcohol. Set aside for several days.

Note that the liquid is full of white particles. The alcohol has coagulated the albumen of the blood.

47. Repeat the last two experiments, using *dilute* alcohol. Note the result after a few days.

Take two bottles, into one of which some days before

were placed weak alcohol and a piece of beef ; into the other, pure alcohol and beef. Take a piece of fresh beef, and you will find that it is as strong as a whip-cord. Now observe these pieces in the bottles. They are dry and brittle. They break like a piece of suet.

48. *To show the Action of Alcohol on Pepsin.* — Take two ordinary wide-mouthed bottles holding from a gill to half a pint (*A* and *B*). Put into the first bottle five grains of pepsin and two or three ounces of lukewarm water. Make it acid with twenty drops of strong muriatic acid.

Do exactly the same thing with the second bottle, except add three tablespoonfuls of alcohol. Set bottles in any convenient place sufficiently warm (near a stove or on a mantel near a warm smoke-pipe) to keep the contents of the bottles at about blood-heat.

After ten hours, note the changes, if any. The pepsin is precipitated in the form of white, stringy particles in the bottle containing alcohol, while the other bottle shows no change ; in other words, the alcohol has precipitated the pepsin of the artificial gastric juice.

49., Prepare the bottles exactly as before. To the bottle *A* add two teaspoonfuls of finely minced albumen. Put it in a warm place, as in Experiment No. 48. Shake very often. The pepsin will begin to act upon the albumen, gradually softening it. In actual digestion, albumen is thus made ready to soak through the moist lining of the stomach.

Do exactly the same thing with the second bottle (*B*), except add three tablespoonfuls of strong alcohol. Expose the bottle to heat, as before. After ten hours, note the result. It will be seen that alcohol has coagulated the albumen in bottle *B*.

50. Repeat Experiment No. 49. Instead of the white

of an egg, add a teaspoonful of finely cut, cooked, and lean beefsteak or corned beef. In the bottle *A* the meat will be more or less dissolved or partially digested in twenty-four hours. In the bottle *B* the effect of the alcohol will be to make the meat seem hard. In short, the alcohol has coagulated the albumen of the meat.

51. Repeat Experiments 48 and 49. Instead of alcohol, use strong beer, whiskey, and rum, to show the action of a more dilute form of alcohol upon the various types of albumen.

52. Repeat Experiment 36. Instead of plain water, add one-quarter of a teaspoonful of common salt to the given amount of water. This saline solution will represent, in a general way, the plasma of the blood. The alcohol will rise in the tube, as in Experiment 36. Now, if we use very dilute alcohol (one part of alcohol to ten parts of water), we find that the alcohol in the tube falls.

In other words, when alcohol is sufficiently dilute, it will go towards the fluid representing the plasma of the blood.

53. *To show how Alcohol coagulates the Blood.* — Get your market-man to carry a clean wide-mouthed fruit-jar to the slaughter-house, and let the butcher fill it with fresh blood. Add at once to the fresh blood a heaping tablespoonful of Epsom salts dissolved in a coffee-cup full of water. This strong saline solution will prevent the formation of a clot. Keep the whole mixture in a cool place, and do not shake it. Draw off two ounces of the mixture, and add to it a pint of water. Set it aside. It remains clear.

Dilute the same amount of the mixture with a pint of water, and pour in a few tablespoonfuls of strong alcohol. Note that the blood is soon coagulated.

54. *To show the Effect of Alcohol on the Blood Corpuscles.* — Squeeze the end of the forefinger, and prick it quick with

a fine needle, drawing a drop of blood. Examine it carefully with a microscope. Note carefully the little corpuscles, their shape, and how they are arranged.

Add the tiniest drop of alcohol. The corpuscles shrink and become of a different or irregular shape. The alcohol has coagulated the albumen of the corpuscles.

55. *To show the Effect of Alcohol on the Circulation of the Blood.* — Stretch the web of a frog's foot over a hole in a thin board, as fully directed in *Our Bodies*, Experiment 72, p. 250. Do this carefully to avoid giving pain to the frog.

Note carefully the circulation of blood through the very small blood-vessels.

Now put on the web a drop of dilute alcohol, and note the result. The little blood-vessels seem to stretch and to allow the blood corpuscles to pass through more rapidly.

The alcohol has weakened the nerves which regulate the flow of blood in the capillaries, thus allowing more blood to flow through them.

56. Repeat the preceding experiment. Instead of dilute, use strong alcohol. Note that the capillaries soon shrivel, and the flow of blood stops.

The alcohol in this case has paralyzed the nerves which control the capillaries. The tiny blood-vessels now contract, and stop the flow of blood.

—

EXPERIMENTS ON DIGESTION

[Chapter VI. page 65.]

57. *To show the Anatomy of Certain Organs, and Parts of Organs, of Digestion.* — Have each pupil examine his own mouth, and also that of some friend. Note the lips, tongue, hard palate, soft palate, uvula, tonsils, and upper part of the gullet.

58. *The Teeth.* — Get a specimen of each kind of tooth if possible. A dentist-friend will give you what you need. Use a very fine saw to saw a perfect molar in two lengthwise. Note its structure in a general way, — its crown, body, cusps, roots, enamel, dentine, pulp-cavity, etc.

59. Make a blackboard sketch of a tooth on a large scale.

Use colored crayon to make plain the various parts.

60. With the help of a mirror, let each pupil locate his own teeth. Note the incisors, eye-teeth, bicuspids, molars, and " wisdom " teeth if any. In the same way, note the teeth of some schoolmate.

61. Locate as near as possible the position of each salivary gland. Press on the part of the cheek opposite the second small molar of the upper jaw,

FIG. 64. — BLACKBOARD SKETCH. Section of a Tooth.

and notice the increased flow of saliva. The appearance of saliva is familiar.

62. *To show Location of Other Organs of Digestion.* — Make a blackboard diagram, in the rough, of the organs of digestion, beginning at the cardiac end of the stomach, after having studied the digestive organs on the chart. Map out on the person in a very general way the location of the stomach, small intestines, and the liver, pancreas, and spleen. The location of the stomach and liver is especially important.

63. *To show how the Wall of the Stomach looks.* — The wall of a pig's stomach resembles the human stomach. Get from the market a piece of the pig's stomach. Cut off bits of it, and examine it thoroughly. Scrape off the inner or

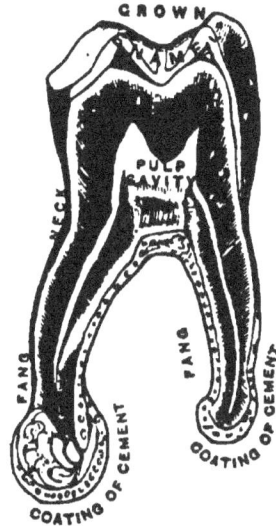

mucous coat with the edge of a very sharp knife. Use a magnifying-glass; find the openings of the gastric tubes. Take a small piece of the wall of the stomach and dissect it with a fine needle, and note the muscular coats.

64. *To show the Action of Saliva.* — Think of some favorite article of food and note the flow of saliva. Push a lead-pencil, or the finger, to and fro in the mouth several times, and note the flow of saliva.

Chew an oyster-cracker, and note carefully how it is moistened with saliva. Grind up several crackers rapidly in the mouth, and note how difficult it is to swallow, or even chew, when there is little saliva.

65. The importance of the saliva in favoring the movements of chewing may be illustrated by the experiment of wiping the inside of the mouth perfectly dry with a towel or handkerchief; when it will be found almost impossible to move the jaws until the saliva is again secreted in sufficient quantity to moisten the surfaces of the tongue, cheeks, and gums.

66. The importance of the saliva as a solvent may be shown by wiping the upper surface of the tongue quite dry with a napkin, and then placing a small quantity of powdered sugar upon it. The sugar will be found to be as destitute of taste as so much sand; whereas in its ordinary moist condition the tongue perceives the taste of sweet substances very distinctly.

This experiment also illustrates the fact that the terminations of the nerves of taste can be affected only by substances brought in contact with them in the liquid state.

67. *To show the Action of Saliva on Starch.* — Chew slowly a piece of fresh bread. Note how sweet it tastes after it is well wet with the saliva. Do the same with a mouthful of paste made of pure arrowroot (almost pure starch), made with boiling water and allowed to cool.

68. *To show the Action of Gastric Juice on Albumen.* — Take an ordinary four-ounce bottle with as wide a mouth as convenient. Put into it the following : Pepsin in scales,[1] one grain, and four tablespoonfuls of lukewarm water. Make it acid with ten drops of strong muriatic acid. Add two teaspoonfuls of finely minced egg-albumen.[2] Set the mixture in any convenient place sufficiently warm, as in a basin of warm water near the stove, or on the mantel near the warm smoke-pipe, to keep the contents of the bottle at about "blood-heat." Shake every few minutes. As soon as the whole mixture becomes of a proper temperature, the pepsin will begin to act upon the albumen which will be gradually softened and digested. This dissolved mass is now in a condition to readily soak through the moist lining of the stomach.

69. Repeat the same experiment, using half a teaspoonful of finely cut, cooked, and lean beefsteak or corned beef instead of the white of an egg.

The meat will be more or less dissolved, or partially digested, in twenty-four hours. This experiment is a crude way to show the action of gastric juice on meat-albumen.

70. *To show the Action of Bile on Fat.* — Shake up a little sweet-oil and water.

"Oil and water will not mix," as the saying goes. Get the butcher to bring you a small bottle of bile (ox-gall), or, better still, ask him to bring the gall-bladder itself. Cut it open, and bottle the contents. Shake up some oil with bile, and a creamy mixture called an " emulsion " results.

---

[1] Pure pepsin is now made by dealers for medical use; and the necessary amount can be bought of a good druggist for a few cents. Use only *pure* pepsin in the experiments.

[2] The albumen or the white of an egg is taken as the *type* of albumen in a naturally pure state, and is well adapted to illustrate the peptonizing action of the gastric ferment. It should be first made ready as follows : Separate the white of a *hard-boiled* egg, and rub it through a coarse sieve, so as to divide it into small particles.

EXPERIMENTS ON THE HEART AND THE CIRCU-
LATION

[CHAPTER VII. PAGE 89.]

EXPERIMENT 71. Tie a string tightly round the finger, and prick the tip of it with a needle. The blood runs freely, is red and opaque. Put a drop of fresh blood on a sheet of clean white paper and note that it looks yellowish.

72. Put a drop of fresh blood on a clean white plate. Cover it with an inverted goblet or sauce-plate. Take off the cover in five minutes, and the drop has set into a jelly-like mass. Breathe into the goblet several times to moisten it, and replace it over the blood. Take it off in half an hour, and a little clot will be seen in the watery serum.

73. To show that blood is really a mass of red bodies, floating in a fluid, which give it the red color. Fill a clean clear glass bottle two-thirds full of little red beads, and then fill the bottle full of water. At a short distance the bottle appears to be filled with a uniformly red liquid.

74. *To find the Pulse.* —With your right hand grasp the right wrist of a friend, pressing with three fingers over the radius. Press three fingers of your right hand over the radius in the left wrist to feel your own pulse. With the aid of a watch,

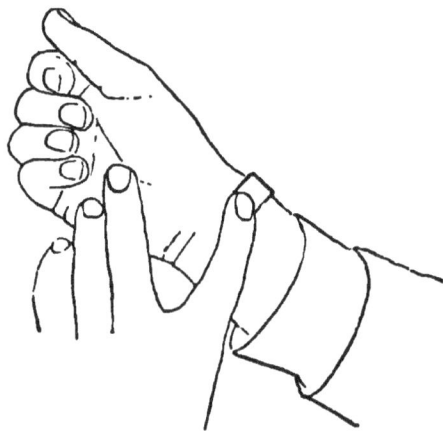

FIG. 65. — How the Pulse may be studied by Mirror on Radial Artery.

count the rate of your own pulse per minute; the same with a friend's pulse.

75. *To show how the Pulse may be studied by pressing a Mirror over the Radial Artery.* — Press a small piece of looking-glass upon the wrist over the radial artery in such a way that with each pulse-beat the mirror may be slightly tilted. If the wrist be now held in such a position that sunlight will fall upon the mirror, a spot of light will be reflected to the opposite side of the room, and by its motion upon the wall will be shown the movements of the artery as the pulse-wave passes through it. — *Bowditch's " Hints for Teachers of Physiology."*

EXPERIMENTS ON THE LUNGS AND BREATHING

[CHAPTER VIII. PAGE 103.]

EXPERIMENT 76. *To locate the Lungs.* — Mark out the boundaries of the lungs by "sounding" them; that is, by percussion as it is called. It simply means, to put one finger across the chest or back, and to give it a quick, sharp rap with another. Note where it sounds hollow; that is, is resonant. This experiment can be done only in a very crude way.

Pupils may be taught to apply their ears to each other's chests in the region of the heart and lungs, and to describe the sounds which they hear. A simple instrument for listening to one's own heart may be made by attaching a piece of rubber tube about eighteen inches long to a small glass funnel.

77. Get a sheep's lungs, with the windpipe attached, from a butcher or marketman. Ask for the heart and lungs in one mass. Take pains to examine the specimen first, and pay

only for a good one.   Parts are apt to be hastily snipped or mangled.

78. Examine the windpipe. Note the horseshoe-shaped rings of gristle in front, which serve to keep it open.

79. Examine one bronchus, carefully dissecting away the lung-tissue with curved scissors. Follow along until small branches of the bronchial tubes are reached. Put pieces of the lung-tissue in a basin of water and see if they float.

80. *To show how the Lung may be filled with Air.* — Take the other lung, and tie a glass tube six inches long into its bronchus. Attach a piece of rubber to one end of the glass tube. Now blow up the lung, and then let it collapse several times. When distended, examine every part of it.

81. *To show that the Air we breathe out is warm.* — Breathe on a thermometer for a few minutes. The mercury will rise rapidly.

82. *To show that it is moist.* — Breathe on a mirror, or a knife-blade, or any polished, metallic surface.

83. *To show that the Air we breathe out contains Carbonic Acid.* — Put a glass tube into a bottle of lime-water, and breathe out into it through the tube. The liquid will soon become cloudy, because the carbonic acid of the expired air throws down the lime held in solution.

84. *To show the Natural Temperature of the Body.* — Borrow a physician's thermometer, and take your own temperature, and that of several friends, by putting it under the tongue, closing the mouth tightly, and holding it there for five minutes.

85. A substitute for a clinical thermometer may be readily contrived by taking an ordinary house thermometer from its tin case and cutting off the lower part of the scale so that the bulb may project freely. With an instrument thus arranged, the pupils may take their own and each

other's temperature; and it will be found that whatever may be the season of the year or the temperature of the room, the thermometer in the mouth will record about 99° F. Care must, of course, be taken to keep the thermometer in the mouth till it ceases to rise, and to read it while it is still in position. —*Prof. H. P. Bowditch.*

EXPERIMENTS ON THE SKIN

[CHAPTER IX. PAGE 116.]

EXPERIMENT 86. *To show the Gross Structure of the Skin.* — Examine your own skin in a general way. Stretch and pull it to show how elastic it is. Get some idea of the scarf skin by scraping off some with a sharp knife. Note any white scars, liver-spots, etc., on the skin. Examine the skin with much care, with the aid of a good magnifying-glass. Note the papillæ on the palm of the hand.

87. *Hair and Nails.* — Pull a stout hair from the head, and examine it carefully with the magnifying-glass. Make a study of the finger-nails.

88. *The Sweat-glands.* — Use a magnifying-glass to study the openings of the sweat-glands, especially on the palms of the hands.

EXPERIMENTS ON THE NERVOUS SYSTEM

[CHAPTER X. PAGE 132.]

EXPERIMENT 89. *Sensations are referred to the Ends of the Nerves.* — Striking the elbow-end of the ulna against anything hard ("hitting the crazy-bone") where the ulna nerve is exposed, the little finger and the ring-finger will tingle, and become numb.

90. *Every Nerve is Independent of any Other.* — Press two fingers closely together. Let the point of the finest needle be carried ever so lightly across from one finger to another, and we can easily tell just when the needle leaves one finger and touches the other.

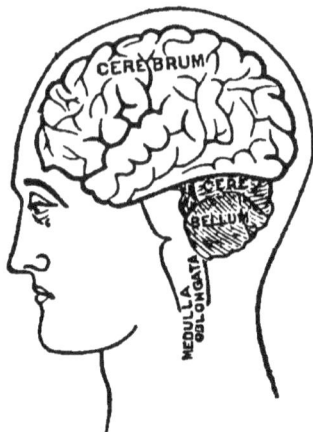

FIG. 66. BLACKBOARD SKETCH.
Showing the Position of the Brain.

91. *One Part of the Body works for the Good of Another Part.* — Tickle the inside of the nose with a feather. This does not interfere at all with the muscles of breathing ; but they come to the help of the irritated part, and provoke a sneeze to clear and protect the nose.

92. *To paralyze a Nerve temporarily.* — Throw one arm over the sharp edge of a chair-back, bringing the inner edge of the biceps directly over the edge of the chair. Press deep and hard for a few minutes. The deep pressure on the nerve of the arm will put the arm " asleep," causing numbness and tingling." The leg and foot often "get asleep" by deep pressure on the nerve of the thigh.

———

EXPERIMENTS ON THE SPECIAL SENSES

[CHAPTER XI. PAGE 153.]

EXPERIMENT 93. Cross the middle finger over the fore-finger, and shut the eyes. Hold a marble between the tips of the crossed fingers. There seems to be two marbles.

94. Shut both eyes, and let a friend run the tips of the fingers first lightly over a hard, plane surface, then pressing hard, and then lightly again, and the surface will seem to be hollowed out.

These two experiments show that we are easily misled, even by the sense of touch. It is mainly matter of habit and education.

95. Put a drop of vinegar on a friend's tongue, or your own. Notice how the papillæ of the tongue start up.

96. Rub different parts of the tongue with the pointed end of a piece of salt and gum-aloes, showing that the *back* of the tongue is most sensitive to salt and bitter substances.

97. Repeat the same with some sweet or sour substances, to show that the *edges* of the tongue are the most sensitive to these things.

98. We often fail to distinguish between the sense of taste and that of smell. Chew some pure, roasted coffee, and it seems to have a distinct taste. Pinch the nose hard, and there is little taste. Coffee has a powerful odor, but only a feeble taste. The same is true of garlic, onions, and various spices.

99. Light helps the sense of taste. Shut the eyes, and palatable foods taste insipid. Pinch the nose, close the eyes, and see how palatable a teaspoonful of cod-liver oil becomes.

100. *The Retina is easily tired.* — With a hand-mirror reflect the sunlight on the white wall, and keep it fixed. Look steadily at it for a full minute, and then let it suddenly be removed. Its " complementary " color — a dark spot — will appear. Pin a round piece of bright red paper (large as a dinner-plate) to a white wall by a single pin. Fasten a long piece of thread to it, so it can be pulled down

in a second. Gaze steadily at the red paper. Have it removed while looking at it intently, and a greenish spot takes its place.

101. *To illustrate the Action of the Crystalline Lens.* — Hold a burning-glass in front of an open window in such a way that the image of some object outside will be brought to a focus upon a piece of paper. This miniature image will be upside down.

102. To vibrate the drum-membrane and the little ear-bones, shut the mouth, and pinch the nose tightly. Try to force air through the nose. The air dilates the eustachian tube, and air is forced into the ear-drum. The distinct crackle, or clicking sound, is due to the movement of the ear-bones and membranes.

103. *The Retina is not sensitive where the Optic Nerve enters the Eyeball.* — This is called the " blind spot." Put two ink-bottles on a table covered over with white paper, about two feet apart. Close the left eye, and fix the right steadily on the left-hand inkstand, gradually varying the distance of the eye to the ink-bottle. At a certain distance the right-hand bottle will disappear ; but, nearer or farther than that, it will be plainly seen.

104. Show the same thing in this way : make two black spots, with pen and ink, as large as two peas, upon a white card, about three inches apart, varying the distance as

FIG. 67. Diagram to show the Existence of the Blind Spot.

before. At a distance of about six inches the "blind spot " will be noticed.

105. *Impressions made upon the Retina do not disappear at*

once. — Look steadily at a bright light for a moment or two, and then turn away suddenly, or shut the eyes. A gleam of light will be seen for a second or two.

106. Take a round piece of white card-board the size of a saucer, and paint it in alternate rings of red and yellow, — two primary colors. Put it on the sewing-machine wheel, or glue it to a grindstone, and rotate it rapidly. The eye perceives neither color, but orange, — the secondary color.

EXPERIMENTS ON THE THROAT AND VOICE

EXPERIMENT 107. *To show the Anatomy of the Throat.* — Study the general construction of the throat by the help of a hand-mirror. Repeat the same on the throat of some friend.

To illustrate the Passage of Air through the Glottis. — Take two strips of india rubber, and stretch them over the open end of a boy's "bean blower," or any kind of a tube. Tie them tightly with thread, so that a chink will be left between them. Force the air through such a tube by blowing hard, and a sound will result if the strips are not too far apart.

EXPERIMENTS ON MATTERS OF EVERY-DAY HEALTH

[CHAPTER XII. PAGE 166.]

EXPERIMENT 108. Imagine a pupil with his fingers or ears frost-bitten. Show how friction should be applied.

Poultices. — Bring a small lot of the necessary material into the schoolroom, and show exactly how a small mustard paste, a flaxseed poultice, or any other simple poultice, is made.

109. *Fainting.* — Select several places about the school-room, and show exactly how a person should be placed, supposing he has fainted in a crowded room. Go through every detail of treatment in your mind.

110. *Apparent Drowning.* — Show exactly how artificial respiration is done. Let a boy lie on a settee, and illustrate the process in every detail. It would be an excellent idea for a teacher to meet his boys at their bathing-place, and show them in still more detail. Let two boys go through the process on a playmate under the eye of the teacher, and then others might follow their example.

111. *Experiments on the Matter of treating Cuts and Bruises, and of stopping Bleeding.* — First, on the matter of treating trifling cuts. Let red-pencil marks made on the face, arms, fingers, etc., stand for cuts. Apply suitable strips of plaster in a proper way for a great variety of imaginary cuts. After putting on the plaster, practise on bandaging the parts with strips of cotton cloth rolled for the purpose. Practise on using the handkerchief for a variety of bandages.

112. *To stop Bleeding from the Arteries.* — Locate the principal arteries on your person and that of a friend. Let red-crayon marks stand for the course of the arteries. Now with strings, cords, shoestrings, handkerchiefs, elastics, strips of clothing, practise tying them so as to press deeply and firmly in the proper place. Let each one in the class practise at the same time on the same artery. Criticise and improve each other's work.

113. *Poisons and their Antidotes.* — Small samples of the more common and important poisons should be shown. Note carefully the appearance of each one. With each sample of poison arrange its most common antidote. Explain exactly how it should be given.

REVIEW ANALYSIS

ALCOHOLIC DRINKS, TOBACCO, AND OTHER NARCOTICS

* The figures in full-face type, in the parentheses, refer to the numbers of the sections in the preceding chapters of this book.

How to Keep Well.

TEST QUESTIONS FOR REVIEW

1. In thinking about our bodies, what questions should we naturally begin to ask?
2. Tell in a general way what this book will try to explain.
3. Tell in your own words some of the good to be got from this study.
4. How may a child get some idea that his body moves?
5. How may a child know that he is warm?
6. How would you compare our bodies to a steam-engine?
7. What happens when the child touches a hot stove, pricks his fingers, or eats some unwholesome fruit?
8. Explain how nerves act somewhat like telegraph-wires.
9. What is the real or essential part of our life?
10. Why is it necessary to know the meaning of certain words at the very beginning of our study?
11. What is meant by anatomy? physiology? hygiene? organ? a tissue? Illustrate.

215

12. What is meant by the function of an organ?
Illustrate.

13. What are glands? Illustrate.

14. What can you say of the general parts of the body?

15. State in a general way the names of the most important organs in the trunk, and locate each one.

16. Why is it a duty to take care of our health?

17. What are some of the ill results of neglecting our health?

THE BONY FRAMEWORK

[CHAPTER II.   PAGE 11.]

1. To what may the bones be compared?

2. What useful purposes do they serve?

3. What do you mean by the skeleton?

4. Describe the composition of bone.

5. Give experiments showing the composition of bone.

6. Explain the general structure of bone.

7. In describing the skeleton, into what divisions will you divide the bones for convenience?

8. Tell what you can about the bones of the head.

9. What can you tell of the dovetailed joints, or sutures?

10. What is meant by the trunk?

11. Tell all you can about the backbone.

12. What are the ribs ?
13. Describe the collar-bone. The shoulder-blade.
14. The bones of the arm. What are they ?
15. Describe the wrist and the fingers.
16. Describe the bones of the leg. The knee-pan.
17. Describe the ankle and the foot.
18. What is a joint ? Mention the different kinds of joints.
19. How are the bones tied to each other ?
20. Give some hints about wearing boots and shoes.
21. What may cause round shoulders and curvature of the spine?
22. What is the effect of alcohol on the bones ?
23. How does tobacco affect the bones ?

THE MUSCLES

[Chapter III. Page 31.]

1. What do muscles enable us to do ?
2. Give some familiar illustrations.
3. Describe the structure of muscle.
4. How do the size and shape of muscles vary ?
5. What peculiar power do muscles have ?
6. Illustrate this power of contraction by a piece of india-rubber.
7. Explain how muscles act to bend the fore-arm.
8. Show how muscles act that are not under the control of the will.
9. Illustrate by the stomach and the heart.

10. What are tendons? Where are they found? What are their uses?
11. Exercise: What is it? Why do we need it?
12. What are some of the advantages of exercise?
13. What is the best time for exercise?
14. Describe the different kinds of exercise.
15. What are the advantages of walking as an exercise? Of light gymnastics?
16. What is the effect of alcohol on the muscles?
17. How does alcohol affect the speech?
18. What is the effect of alcohol on the strength?
19. What proofs have we of this effect of alcohol?
20. What can you say of the effect of tobacco on the muscles?

WHAT WE EAT AND DRINK

[CHAPTER IV.   PAGE 46.]

1. To illustrate work, waste, and repair, how may you compare the body to a steam-engine? Explain fully.
2. Why do we need food?
3. What is meant by the tissue foods?
4. Give some familiar examples.
5. What are the sugars and starches? Give examples.
6. Describe the fats and illustrate.
7. What is meant by the mineral foods?
8. Illustrate the value of salt as a food.
9. What can you say of water as a food?

10. Give in detail the more important articles of diet.
11. In a general way what can you say of artificial drinks?
12. What are some of the more common artificial drinks?
13. What can you say of the effect of drinking tea?
14. How does coffee affect the health?
15. Mention some of the ill effects of drinking too much ice-water.

ORIGIN AND NATURE OF FERMENTED DRINKS

[CHAPTER V. PAGE 56.]

1. What is meant by sweet apple-juice?
2. What change takes place soon after it is pressed out?
3. What causes the change in the pressed-out fruit-juices?
4. What is meant by a ferment?
5. Where are the ferments before the apples are ground?
6. What effect has warmth on a ferment?
7. Give a definition of alcohol.
8. Mention the main points of contrast between alcohol and water.
9. What is meant by the alcohol appetite?
10. How does it differ from a natural appetite?
11. What proves the strength of the alcoholic appetite?

12. To what is drunkenness due?
13. Why should not alcohol be used as a flavoring in cooking?
14. What is vinous fermentation?
15. What is the law of fermentation?
16. How is this illustrated when cider changes to vinegar?
17. Tell of some of the evils of cider-drinking.
18. Explain how wine is made.
19. How may we know there is alcohol in wine?
20. What changes the nature of the grape-juice when wine is made?
21. In what does this change consist?
22. Why is wine a dangerous drink?
23. Illustrate by its use in foreign lands.
24. Explain how beer is made.
25. Show how the law of fermentation applies to the process of beer-making.
26. What are the dangers in drinking beer?
27. How does beer-drinking give a false appearance of health?
28. What can you say of beer-drinking from a moral point of view?
29. Show how bread is made by fermentation.
30. What is meant by distilled liquors?
31. Mention some of the more common distilled liquors.
32. Why are they so destructive to health?

DIGESTION AND HOW IT GOES ON

[CHAPTER VI. PAGE 65.]

1. Explain how food is made ready to mix with the blood.
2. What is meant by digestion?
3. Describe the two sets of teeth.
4. Tell something about the structure of a tooth.
5. What takes place in the mouth during digestion?
6. What is the saliva? and what is its action?
7. Describe the process of swallowing.
8. What prevents the food from going into the windpipe?
9. Tell what you can about the stomach.
10. What is the gastric juice, and what is its action?
11. What can you tell of Alexis St. Martin?
12. What is meant by the intestines?
13. Tell what you can about the liver.
14. In what two ways is the nutritious part of food taken into the blood?
15. What is meant by absorption?
16. Explain the action of the lacteals.
17. What is the thoracic duct?
18. What are the lymphatics, and what do they do?
19. *How much* should we eat?
20. What general rules to guide as to *what* we should eat?
21. Describe in some detail *when* we should eat.
22. Explain in a general way *how* we should eat.
23. Why is the proper cooking of food a matter of great importance?

24. Give what hints you can about the care of the teeth.
25. What is the effect of alcohol on digestion in the stomach?
26. How does alcohol affect the liver?
27. What is the effect of tobacco on digestion?

THE BLOOD, THE RIVER OF LIFE

[CHAPTER VII.   PAGE 89.]

1. How does blood look to the naked eye?
2. Is it really red?
3. What gives it its red color?
4. Illustrate by some familiar thing.
5. Describe the blood corpuscles.
6. Give some familiar illustrations to show their size.
7. What do you mean by fibrine? serum? clot?
8. What is meant by the circulation of blood?
9. What can you tell of Dr. Harvey and his discovery?
10. What is an artery? a vein? a capillary?
11. Describe the heart.
12. What is meant by auricle? ventricle? aorta?
13. Describe in detail the circulation of a drop of blood, starting from the left auricle
14. What can you say, in a general way, of the work done by the heart?
15. What is the pulse? What does it tell us?
16. What is the effect of exercise on the circulation?

17. How may the heart be injured by violent effort ?
18. How does tight clothing affect the circulation ?
19. In what two ways does alcohol get into the blood ?
20. What effect does alcohol have on the circulation ?
21. Explain the action of alcohol on the heart.
22. What is the effect of tobacco on the heart ?

HOW AND WHY WE BREATHE

[CHAPTER VIII. PAGE 103.]

1. What is meant by breathing ?
2. What is it that we breathe ? Give some familiar illustrations.
3. Describe the lungs.
4. What can you tell about the windpipe ?
5. Show how the voice is produced.
6. Describe the inner structure of the lungs.
7. Define inspiration ; expiration ; respiration.
8. Describe in detail the process of breathing.
9. Tell something about the work of the diaphragm.
10. What is meant by oxygen and nitrogen ?
11. Describe in detail what takes place in the lungs.
12. Mention the most important changes in the air from breathing.
13. Tell what you can about carbonic-acid gas and its poisonous effects.
14. How is the air kept pure ?
15. How is the air we breathe made impure ? about the house ? in various trades ?

16. Why and how should we ventilate? Give some practical plans.
17. What can you say of the ventilation of bedrooms?
18. Explain the effect of alcohol upon the air-passages.
19. How does tobacco affect the air-passages?

HOW OUR BODIES ARE COVERED

[CHAPTER IX. PAGE 116.]

1. In what three ways does the body get rid of its waste matter?
2. The true skin; describe its structure.
3. Describe the structure of the scarf-skin.
4. What is the sweat? and where does it come from?
5. Why do we need to wash ourselves?
6. Describe the hair and the nails.
7. What gives the hair its color? Give some illustrations.
8. What will cause the hair to change its color?
9. What care should be taken of the nails?
10. Baths; why, when, and how should they be taken?
11. How is the body kept warm? Explain in detail.
12. How is the heat of the body regulated?
13. Why do we need clothing?
14. Give some hints about the use of clothing.
15. Describe the effect of alcohol upon the bodily heat.

16. What effect does alcohol have upon the power of the body to endure extremes of heat or cold?

17. How does tobacco affect the skin?

THE NERVOUS SYSTEM

[CHAPTER X. PAGE 132.]

1. Show how the different parts of the body act in harmony.

2. What is meant by the nervous system? and what are its parts?

3. Tell what you can about the brain.

4. What can you say of the spinal cord and the nerves?

5. How would you compare the nervous system to the telegraph?

6. Give some familiar illustrations.

7. Describe in detail what is meant by reflex action.

8. Show the importance of reflex action.   Illustrate.

9. What can you say about the importance of keeping the nervous system in good health?

10. What is sleep?   Show how necessary it is to health.

11. Give some practical hints about getting proper sleep.

12. What is the first result after alcohol is taken?

13. What is the effect of alcohol on the brain?

14. How does alcohol affect the judgment?

15. What is the effect of alcoholic liquors on the will?

16. To what disease of the nervous system may alcohol finally lead?
17. Show how the craving for alcohol may be inherited.
18. What can you say of the use of tobacco?
19. What is the effect of its continued use?
20. Why is tobacco especially hurtful to young people?
21. What will you say of cigarettes, and the harm they do?
22. What can you say of the use of tobacco, from a moral point of view?
23. What is opium? Describe the opium habit.
24. Give some practical points about opium.
25. What can you say of the chloral habit?

THE FIVE GATEWAYS OF KNOWLEDGE

[CHAPTER XI. PAGE 153.]

1. What is meant by the "five gateways of knowledge"?
2. Name the five special senses.
3. Describe the sense of touch.
4. Tell what you can about the sense of taste.
5. To what extent may this sense be cultivated?
6. Describe the sense of smell.
7. Tell what you can about the outer ear.
8. Describe the middle ear.
9. Tell something about the inner ear.
10. Give some practical hints about the care of the ear.

11. What can you say of the great importance of sight ?
12. Describe the general structure of the eye.
13. Show how the eye is protected.
14. What is meant by color-blindness ?
15. Show how it is a matter of practical importance.
16. How would you take good care of your eyes ?
17. Describe the effect of alcohol on the special senses.
18. What effect does tobacco have on the special senses ?

WHAT TO DO IN ACCIDENTS AND ILLNESS

[CHAPTER XII. PAGE 166.]

1. Mention some accidents and emergencies likely to occur any day.
2. What would you do for a fainting person ?
3. What is the treatment for frostbite ?
4. Describe fits, and tell what to do for them.
5. What is suffocation ? What would you do for it ?
6. What can you say about broken bones ?
7. What is the treatment for the sting of insects ? for nosebleed ?
8. What would you do for a foreign body in the nose ? in the ear ? in the throat ? in the eye ?
9. What is the treatment for sunstroke or heatstroke ?
10. What would you do for burns or scalds ?

11. What can you say of bruises? of cut and torn wounds?
12. How would you stop bleeding from an artery? from a vein?
13. Describe in detail how you would manage a case of apparent drowning.
14. Give some hints about the proper care of the bowels.
15. What can you say of the habit of taking unknown medicines?
16. Give in detail how you would take care of a sick-room.
17. Mention the various ways in which the air may be poisoned from diseases that spread.
18. What is meant by disinfection?
19. What can you tell in a general way of poisons?
20. What golden rule can you give concerning poisons?

NOTES

Note 1. — " If by the aid of the microscope we examine a very fine section of muscle taken from a person in good health, we find the muscle firm, elastic, and of a bright red color, made up of parallel fibres with beautiful crossings or striæ; but if we similarly examine the muscle of a man who leads an idle, sedentary life, and indulges in intoxicating drinks, we detect at once a pale, flabby, inelastic, oily appearance." — *Dr. Henry Monroe.*

" It [alcohol] greatly lessens muscular tone and power. There is no evidence that it increases nervous influence, while there is much evidence that it lessens nervous power." — *Dr. E. Smith in Philosophical Transactions for* 1859.

" I found that alcohol weakens the muscular contraction and lessens the time during which the contraction can continue active." — *Dr. B. W. Richardson.*

Note 2. — "A soldier was experimented upon by being given a certain amount of work to do, first when his system was free from the effects of alcohol, and second when under the influence of certain measured doses of brandy. The result is summed up as follows: The brandy seemed to give him a kind of spirit which made him think he could do a great deal of work, but when he came to do it he found he was less capable than he thought. The experience of this man harmonizes with the advice that is given by guides and others who are in the habit of ascending mountains. Spirits, they say, take away the strength from the legs, and should therefore be avoided during a fatiguing expedition." — *F. W. Pavy in "Food and Dietetics."*

"It was quite remarkable to observe how much stronger and more able to do their work the men were when they had nothing but water to drink." — *Sir John Ross in an account of his Arctic explorations.*

The Army of the Potomac, in the spring of 1862, was subjected to great hardships in labor, and exposed to the extremely wet and malarious region of the Chickahominy. There was, consequently, much sickness and suffering. Under these circumstances the commanding general issued an order on the 19th of May, allowing every officer and soldier one gill of whiskey per day, half to be served in the morning and half in the evening. The results were so manifestly injurious to the sanitary condition of the army that in just thirty days the order was countermanded by the same general. Concerning this experiment in the Army of the Potomac, Dr. Frank Hamilton, one of the most eminent surgeons serving with that army, says : "It is earnestly desired that no such experiment will ever be repeated in the armies of the United States."

The following story was told by a sea-captain to a lady whose name is a household word in many parts of this country : —

"When I was yet a lad before the mast I had a memorable adventure. It was winter, and we were off a rocky lee-shore with a tremendous storm upon us. We tacked off and on, and with every tack we had to break the icicles off the ropes, it was so fearfully cold. Of course one of the first things was to serve out gin. This made the men work well a little while after each drink, and then they would flag and call for more gin. Gradually they grew worse, and finally they could not be made to work at all. Before morning every one of them was laid up and helpless. I did not drink, and there were two lads with me whom I persuaded not to drink. At last we were the only ones who were able to do anything, and it was all we could do to keep the vessel on her way until the storm abated." — " And what if you had drunk with the rest ? " he was asked. " We should all have gone to the bottom together ; no possible help for it," he replied.

NOTE 3. — " The idea that tobacco gives increased power to endure either physical or mental hardships is one of the greatest delusions of the age. Tobacco and alcohol, though unlike in many respects, have many points of resemblance, and arguments against one are usually valid against the other. Both are poisons, and both are regarded by many as necessities. It was formerly thought that alcohol augmented strength, but it has been found by experiments that the man who drinks it cannot lift so heavy a weight as those who do not, though he feels as if he could lift a much heavier one. Tobacco may for a short time make a man less conscious of his fatigue ; but the truth is that his strength is diminished rather than increased by its use." — *Thomas G. Roberts, M. D.*

" The winning boat of Harvard University, and the loosing boat of Yale, were not rowed by smokers. One of the first things demanded of a young man who is going into training for a boat race is, stop smoking. And he himself, long before his body has reached its highest point of purity and development, will become conscious of the lowering and disturbing effects of smoking one inch of a mild cigar. No smoker who has ever trained severely for a race, or a game, needs to be told that smoking reduces the tone of his system and diminishes all the forces of his body. He knows it.

He has been as conscious of it as a boy is of the effects of his first cigar." —*James Parton.*

" Its [tobacco's] power of causing relaxation of the muscular system is great." — *Appleton's Cyclopædia, vol. xii. p.* 784.

NOTE 4. — " Alcohol is classed among the poisons by medical writers on poisons. I do not know of an exception among physicians. It is ranked among the poisons from its effects on the body analogous to those of the other poisons. What is said of the effect of alcohol must be true of all doses, large or small, although the effect of very minute doses may be imperceptible. Arsenic may be administered in doses so small as to produce no apparent ill effects; yet no one doubts that arsenic is a poison. . . . If a person dies of delirium tremens it is not the last glass that kills him, but every dose or glass he has taken in his life has conduced to the result." — *Dr. Reuben D. Mussey, Professor of Anatomy and Surgery, Dartmouth College.*

" We believe that alcohol is ever a poison." — *Editor of the Revue Scientifique of France.*

" Alcohol is universally ranked among poisons by physiologists, chemists, physicians, toxicologists, and all who have experimented, studied, and written upon the subject, and who, therefore, best understand it. It is not necessary to the action of poisons that they be always swallowed in fatal doses." — *Professor W. J. Youmans, in his work on Alcohol.*

" Is alcohol a poison? I reply, yes. It answers to the description of a poison. It possesses an inherent, deleterious property, which, when introduced into the system, is capable of destroying life, and it has its place with arsenic, bella-donna, prussic acid, opium, etc. Toxicologists divide poisons into three classes : Irritants, Narcotics, and Narcotico-Irritants. Alcohol belongs to the latter class. In its effects upon the living system it is first an irritant, and afterward when it has entered the circulation it becomes a narcotic. Were alcohol an irritant only, a man would as soon poison himself with arsenic or aquafortis. The narcotic element is the Siren that leads him on to ruin and to death." — *Dr. Willard Parker.*

NOTE 5.— Professor W. F Wessen, who resided seven years in beer-drinking Germany, said of the students in the universities of Berlin and Halle, " One-third of the students are once a week what you would call drunk. As regards the people, I can only say that during the last five years drunken people have gone past my house, I suppose, every evening, sometimes boisterously drunk and sometimes reelingly drunk."

The *Reichanzeiger*, of Berlin, published, Oct. 7, 1891, in full, the Emperor's proposed law against the " abuse of spirituous liquors," and presented in a long article of nearly eleven columns the reason for its passage. Among these were the following : " The intemperate use of spirits increases the mortality, causes many cases of sickness, is the fountain of pauperism, undermines morality, and ruins the family life. The cases of chronic alcoholism and delirium tremens in Germany, which have been treated in public institutions, have increased from 4,272 in 1877 to 10,360 in 1885. Among the latter number were 673 females.

Still clearer is the percentage of such cases treated when compared with other patients. The alcoholic cases furnish nearly twenty per cent of all the cases treated in the public hospitals. The insane asylums received 1,161 patients in 1885 ; 1,213 men and 121 women died of delirium tremens in 1886. Of the prisoners in German penitentiaries convicted of murder, forty-six per cent used liquor, and of these again forty-one per cent were habitual drunkards. Of those who committed manslaughter, sixty-three per cent were drinkers. Violent assaults were in seventy-four per cent of the cases committed by drunkards, and the other crimes varied from forty to sixty-eight per cent.

NOTE 6. — " The diseases of beer-drinkers are always of a dangerous character, and in the case of an accident, they can never undergo the most trifling operation with the security of the temperate." — *Dr. Edwards.*

NOTE 7. — " Alcohol inflames the stomach, weakens the power of digestion and assimilation, and cannot be long continued without disastrous results. . . . It takes but a small quantity of alcohol to inflame the stomach and brain of persons who have not been accustomed to its use." — *Dr. R. Greene.*

" I support the statement of the late Dr. Cheyne that nothing more effectually hinders digestion than alcohol. I hold that those who abstain from alcohol have the best digestion; and that more instances of indigestion, of flatulency, of acidity, and of depression of mind and body, are produced by alcohol than by any other single cause." — *Dr. B. W. Richardson.*

" Alcohol is a poison forever at war with man's nature, and in all its forms and degrees of strength produces irritation of the stomach, which is liable to result in inflammation, ulceration, and mortification, a thickening and indurating of its coats; and finally malignant cancer, and other organic affections; and it may be asserted with confidence that no one who indulges habitually in the use of alcoholic drinks, whether in the form of wine or more ardent spirits, possesses a healthy stomach." — *Dr. Thomas Sewell, Professor of Pathology and Practice of Medicine in Columbia College, D. C.*

NOTE 8.—" The organ of the body most frequently injured by the use of alcohol is the liver. As in poisoning by arsenic, strychnine, and other such drugs, it is found that the liver is the place where they are mostly deposited; so it is with alcohol. The liver of the confirmed drunkard is probably never entirely free from its influence and is often fairly saturated with it.* The action of alcohol upon the liver is similar to its action upon the stomach. It first becomes enlarged, and its activity is increased, and then it becomes shrunken, hardened, and roughened, and its' action is perverted and decreased. It, in some cases, looks as if it had been driven full of round-headed nails. Hence it has received the name of 'hob-nailed liver' or 'gin-drinker's liver.'" — *Dr. D. A. Robinson.*

NOTE 9. — " 'The effects of tobacco on the stomach are twofold and arise from two distinct poisons. . . . The bitter extract which so readily excites vomiting in the young smoker appears to act at all times with more or less violence on the mucous lining. At first it produces great irritation and redness. After a time these changes are subdued, but are not entirely removed. The membrane secretes irregularly, and, as a general rule, does not produce the due amount of gastric fluid; hence, digestion is impeded. After digestion an acrid fluid is left in the stomach, which irritates and gives rise to heartburn, eructations, frequent nausea with an almost constant sensation of debility of the stomach, and sometimes to cravings for particular foods, especially for those that have an acid reaction, such as pickles and fresh fruit.

" The muscular portion of the stomach is acted upon by

the nicotine. In small quantities the nicotine excites a slight movement in the muscular fibres. . . . Carried to excess it produces a palsied condition of the muscular fibres, leading to increased debility in the digestive organs, to a serious impairment of their functions, and to constipation.

"So long as the digestive organs are functionally disturbed, so long the whole of the body, looking to them as it does for the sources of supply, is held, proportionally, in want and exhaustion. If at the same time waste were not to a certain extent prevented, that exhaustion would soon be increased even to danger." — *Dr. B. W. Richardson.*

"A professor connected with a prominent medical college. while lecturing on disorders of the liver, stated that the use of tobacco in even the smallest amount impairs the functional action of the liver on the blood passing through it and that the abnormal state of the blood thus caused will manifest itself by disturbance in the brain." — Quoted by C. W. Lyman in an article on Tobacco in the *New York Medical Journal,* Sept. 8, 1888.

NOTE 10.—"The vessels of the lungs are easily relaxed by alcohol ; and as they of all parts are most exposed to vicissitudes of heat and cold, they are readily congested when, paralyzed by the spirits, they are subjected to the effects of a sudden fall of atmospheric temperature : thus the sudden fatal congestions of the lungs which so easily befall the confirmed alcoholic during severe winter seasons." — *Dr. B. W. Richardson.*

"There can be no question but that inhalation of smoke induces disease of the mucous membrane with which it comes in contact ; it will produce a catarrhal state of the nose and throat where none exists, and it may awaken a new one in a patient who has been cured of the disease. It may produce a cancerous tumor of the throat or tongue, which may become very serious." — *Dr. Orlando Mixter.*

"Tobacco causes irritation of the mucous membrane of the mouth and throat, more especially in the case of cigarette smoking." — *Dr. E. O. Otis.*

NOTE 11. — The *Cincinnati Medical Repertory*, in a recent article, gives an account of a company of twenty-six men who were travelling across a western plain and lost their way as night came on. The weather was intensely cold, and they had no means of making a fire. They had each two blankets, plenty of food and whiskey. This last they were advised by the leader of the party not to take, but to eat a good supper and wrap themselves up in their blankets and lie close together. Two besides himself heeded his advice ; and, though they were cold, they did not suffer nor freeze. Three others drank a very little. They suffered greatly, but were not frozen. Seven others who drank considerable had their toes and fingers frozen, but got over it in a few weeks. Six who drank still more were badly frozen and never got over it. Four who got intoxicated were so bady frozen that they died in a few weeks, while three who got dead drunk were found dead in the morning. Thus all who drank the whiskey suffered in proportion to the amount they drank.

NOTE 12. — "Alcohol, when taken in small quantity, is in general said to act as a direct cardiac stimulant, and its stimulating effect is supposed to be due to its possessing the faculty of increasing the muscular power of the heart. I take an entirely different view of the matter, and shall endeavor to show how the increase in the force of the heart's movement, the quickening of the pulse, the flushing of the face, the congestion of the retinal blood-vessels, as well as

all the other visible appearances of accelerated cardiac functional activity are in reality in no wise due to the stimulating
action of alcohol, either on the heart's muscular tissue or the
nerves supplying it, but actually to the very reverse, namely,
its paralyzing effect on the cardiac nerve mechanism." — *Dr.
George Harley, in London Lancet, March,* 1888.

Dr. James Barr, of the Northern Hospital, London, in a
clinical lecture reported in the *London Lancet,* January, 1881,
said that Dr. Samuel Wilkes over twenty years ago " showed
that alcohol was not a stimulant in the proper sense of the
term, but a sedative " [or narcotic], and that "not one word "
of what Dr. Wilkes then stated "had ever been since seriously controverted and, certainly, never disproved."

" In general, let it be understood that all the workings of
alcohol in the system which usually are considered as excitement or stimulation are only the indications of paralysis." —
*Prof. G. Bunge, of the Chair of Physiological Chemistry in the
University of Basle, Switzerland.*

" Alcohol has clearly no right to be called a stimulant. It
is a narcotic from first to last." — *Dr. J. J. Ridge, England.*

As long ago as 1830, Dr. Beaumont, who made the celebrated " Observations " on the stomach of Alexis St. Martin,
said, " The whole class of alcoholic liquors may be considered as narcotics, producing very little difference in their
ultimate effects on the system."

Dr. John Higginbottom, F.R.S., after more than fifty
years of practice, said, " Alcohol is neither food nor physic,
for alcohol, in all its forms, instead of nourishing, poisons ;
instead of strengthening, it weakens ; instead of stimulating,
it narcotizes and paralyzes ; instead of increasing the vital
forces, it diminishes force, produces disease, and is an agent
of degeneration and death."

NOTE 13. — "The more purely intellectual qualities of the mind rarely escape being involved in the general disturbance. The power of application, of appreciating the bearings of facts, of drawing distinctions, of exercising the judgment aright, and even of comprehension, are all more or less impaired. The sense of right and justice which the individual may have had is so weakened or destroyed that he will lie, steal, murder, or commit other outrages, even when there is no provocation. . . . The perceptions, the emotions, the intellect, and the will are all implicated to a greater or less degree." — *Dr. William A. Hammond, in Diseases of the Nervous System.*

NOTE 14. — A document published by the Legislature of the State of New York, entitled "The Twentieth Annual Report of the Prison Association of New York," contains the following record : " There can be no doubt that of all the proximate sources of crime the use of intoxicating liquors is the most prolific and the most deadly. Of other causes it may be said that they slay their thousands ; of this it may be acknowledged that it slays its tens of thousands. The Committee asked for the opinion of the jail officers in nearly every county of the State as to the proportion of commitments due either directly or indirectly to strong drink. The judgment of these jail officers varied from two-thirds, the lowest estimate, to nine-tenths as the highest, and on reducing the several proportions to the average, seven-eighths was the result obtained."

"I have practised law for forty years, have been engaged in over four thousand criminal cases, and on mature reflection I am convinced that more than three thousand of them originated in drunkenness alone, and that a great proportion of the remainder could be traced either directly or indirectly to this source." — *Hon. A. B. Richmond.*

When the Hon. E. C. Delevan, of Albany, was in Rome, Cardinal Acton, the Supreme Judge, assured him that nearly all the crime in Rome originated in the use of wine.

NOTE 15. — " The hereditary influence of alcohol manifests itself in various ways. It transmits an appetite for strong drink to the children, and these are likely to have that form of drunkenness which may be termed paroxysmal; that is, they will go for a considerable period without indulging, placing restraint upon themselves, but at last all the barriers of self-control give way; they yield to the irresistible appetite, and then their indulgence is extreme. The drunkard by inheritance is a more helpless slave than his progenitor; and the children that he begets are more helpless still, unless upon the mother's side there is ingrafted upon them untainted stock. But its hereditary influence is not confined to the propagation of drunkards. It produces insanity, idiocy, epilepsy, and other affections of the brain and nervous system, not only in the transgressor himself, but in his children, and these will transmit predisposition to any of these diseases. . . . When alcoholism does not produce insanity, idiocy, or epilepsy, it weakens the conscience, impairs the will, and makes the individual the creature of impulse and not of reason." — *Dr. Willard Parker.*

" The appetite for strong drink is frequently transmitted from parents to the children, just as other traits of the mind or body. Sometimes it develops early, sometimes late in life ; as a rule, this hereditary propensity shows itself at an early age, and is apt to be intensified at the age of maturity."— *Dr. James C. Wilson, in Pepper's System of Medicine, Vol. v., p.* 634.

NOTE 16. — " Tobacco deranges the whole nervous system."— *Dr. B. W. Richardson.*

"Tobacco reduces the intellectual power of a boy. It does this either by opposing mental application and effort, or else by producing deterioration of the intellect, probably both to a greater or less degree." — *Dr. Edward O. Otis, in Boston Medical and Surgical Journal.*

"I believe the use of tobacco by cadets induces difficulty of concentrating the mind upon study." — *Medical Inspector Gorgas, of the U. S. Naval Academy.*

"Smoking tobacco weakens the nervous powers, favors a dreamy, imaginative, and imbecile state of mind, produces indolence and incapacity for manly or continuous exertion, and sinks its votary into a state of careless or maudlin inactivity and selfish enjoyment of his vice." — *Dr. J. Copeland, F.R.S.*

"It is our deliberate opinion that the unsatisfactory recitations and consequent failures at final examination, so injurious to the interests of this establishment, are to be attributed, in great measure, to nervous derangement caused by the common use of tobacco by the students. It becomes our duty to recommend some stringent measures to correct this practice."—*Medical Report on the Use of Tobacco by the Cadets at the U. S. Naval Academy.*

GLOSSARY

Ab-do'men. See Sect. 6.

Ab-sorp'tion. The process of sucking up nutritive or waste matters by the blood-vessels.

A'cid. A substance usually sour, sharp, or biting to the taste.

Ad'am's Ap'ple. An angular projection of cartilage in the front of the neck. .

Al-bu'men. An animal substance resembling the white of an egg.

A-nat'o-my. See Sect. 5.

A-or'ta. The largest artery of the body. .

A'que-ous Humor. The watery fluid occupying the space between the cornea and crystalline lens of the eye.

Ar'ter-y. A vessel by which blood is carried from the heart.

Au'di-to-ry Nerve. The special nerve of hearing.

Au'ri-cle. A cavity of the heart.

Bile. The gall; a secretion of the liver.

Bronch'i. The first two branches of the windpipe.

Bronch'i-al Tubes. The smaller branches of the windpipe.

Ca-nal'. In the body, any tube or passage.

Cap'il-la-ry. The " hair-like " blood-vessels.

Car-bon'ic A'cid. The gas which is breathed out from the lungs; a waste product of the animal kingdom, and a food of the vegetable kingdom.

Car-di'ac. The orifice of the stomach, near the heart.

Car'ron Oil. A mixture of equal parts of linseed-oil and lime water.

Car'ti-lage. A tough but flexible material, forming a part of the joints, nostrils, ears ; gristle.

Ca'se-ine. The albumen part of milk ; forming the basis of cheese.

Cer-e-bel'lum. The little brain.

Cer'e-brum. The brain proper.

Chlo'ral. A powerful drug used by physicians to induce sleep.

Cir-cu-la'tion. The course of the blood through the blood-vessels of the body.

Co-ag-u-la'tion. Applied to the process by which the blood clots or becomes solid.

Con-ges'tion. An unnatural gathering of blood in any part of the body.

Con-sti-pa'tion. Costiveness ; tardiness in evacuating the bowels.

Con-vul'sion. A more or less violent agitation of the limbs or body; a fit.

Corn. A portion of the outer skin, of horn-like hardness.

Cor'ne-a. The transparent substance which covers a part of the front of the eyeball.

Cor'pus-cles, Blood. The small bodies which give to the blood its red color.

Crys'tal-line Lens. A double-convex body situated in the front part of the eyeball.

Cu'ti-cle. The scarf-skin ; also called the *epider'mis.*

Cu'tis. The true skin, lying beneath the cuticle ; also called the *der'mis.*

De-lir'i-um. A state in which the ideas of a person are wild, irregular, and unconnected.

Di'a-phragm. See Sect. 6.

Dis-in-fect'ants. Agents used to destroy the causes of infection.

Dis'til-la'tion. Consult Webster's International Dictionary.

Duct. A canal or tube.

Dys-pep'si-a. Indigestion.

El'e-ment. One of the simplest parts of which anything consists.

E-met'ic. A medicine which causes vomiting.

E-mul'sion. Oil in a finely divided state, suspended in water.

En-am'el. The dense material which covers the crown of a tooth.

Ep-i-glot'tis. See Sect. 55.

Ex-cre'tion. The separation from the blood, of the waste matters of the body.

Ex-pi-ra't:on. The act of forcing air out of the lungs.

Ex-ten'sion. The act of restoring a limb, etc., to its natural position after it has been flexed.

Fer'ment. Consult Webster's International Dictionary.

Fer'men-ta'tion. See " Ferment."

Fi'bre. One of the tiny threads of which many parts of the body are composed.

Fi'brine. A substance like albumen, found in the blood.

Flex'ion. The act of bending a limb.

Func'tion. The special duty of any organ of the body.

Gas'tric. Pertaining to the stomach.

Gel'a-tine. An animal substance which dissolves in hot water, and forms a jelly on cooling.

Germ. A living particle detached from already existing living matter.

Gland. See Sect. 5.

Glu'ten. The albumen-like part of wheat.

Gym-nas'tics. The practice of athletic exercises.

Hy'gi-ene. See Sect. 5.

In-spi-ra'tion. The act of drawing in the breath.

In-tes'tines. The bowels.

I'ris. The thin curtain between the cornea and crystalline lens, giving the eye its color.

Lac'te-als. The absorbent vessels of the small intestines.

Lig'a-ment. A strong, fibrous material, binding bones or other parts together.

Mar'row. The soft, fatty substance contained in bones.

Mas-ti-ca'tion. Act of chewing.

Mi'cro-scope. An optical instrument which assists in the examination of minute objects.

Mu'cous Mem'brane. The thin layer of tissue which covers those parts which communicate with the external air.

Mu'cus. The glairy fluid which is secreted by mucous membranes, serving to keep them in a moist condition.

Nar-cot'ic. A drug which in sufficient doses produces stupor, convulsions, and sometimes death.

Na'sal. Pertaining to the nose.

Nic'o-tine. The poisonous oil extracted from tobacco.

Nos'trils. The two outer openings of the nose.

Nu-tri'tion. The processes by which the nourishment of the body is accomplished.

Ol-fac'to-ry. Pertaining to the sense of smell.

Op'tic. Pertaining to the sense of sight.

Or'bit. The bony socket in which the eyeball is situated.

Or'gan. A portion of the body having some special duty.

Pal-pi-ta'tion. A violent and irregular beating of the heart.

Pa-pil'la. The name of the small elevations found on the skin and mucous membranes.

Pa-ral'y-sis. Loss of motion or feeling; palsy.

Pep'sin. The active principle of the gastric juice.

Per-spi-ra'tion. The sweat.

Pha-lan'ges. The bones of the fingers and toes.

Phys-i-ol'o-gy. See Sect. 5.

Plas'ma. The liquid part of the blood.

Poi'son. Any substance which, when applied externally, or taken into the stomach or the blood, produces disease or death.

Pul'mo-na-ry. Pertaining to the lungs.

Pulse. See Sect. 74.

Pu'pil. The opening in the iris through which light passes into the eye.

Py-lo'rus. The outlet from the stomach into the small intestine.

Re'flex. The name given to certain involuntary movements.

Res-pi-ra'tion. Breathing.

Ret'i-na. The innermost of the coats of the eyeball, being an expansion of the optic nerve.

Sa-li'va. The spittle.

Se-cre'tion. The process of separating from the blood some essential fluid, which is also called a secretion.

Sen-sa'tion. The perception of an external impression by the nervous system.

Se'rum. The clear, watery fluid which separates from the clot of the blood.

Sock'et. An opening into which anything is fitted.

Spasm. A sudden, violent, and involuntary contraction of one or more muscles.

Spe'cial Sense. A sense by which we receive particular sensations, such as those of sight, hearing, taste, and smell.

Sprain. An injury to the ligaments or tendons about a joint.

Stim'u-lant. An agent which causes an increase of vital activity in the body or any of its parts.

Sut'ure. The union of certain bones of the skull by the interlocking of jagged edges.

Ten'don. The white, fibrous cord, by which a muscle is attached to a bone ; a sinew.

Tho'rax. The chest.

Tis'sue. See Sect. 5.

To-bac'co. A plant used for smoking and chewing, and in snuff.

Tra'che-a. The windpipe.

Vein. A vessel by which blood is carried to the heart.

Ven-ti-la'tion. The introduction of fresh air into a room or building in such a manner as to keep pure the air within.

Ven'tri-cles of the Heart. The two largest cavities of the heart.

Ver'te-bra. One of the bones which make the backbone.

Ver'te-bral Col'umn. The backbone ; also called the spinal column, and spine.

Vil'li. Minute thread-like projections found upon the inner surface of the small intestine, giving it an appearance like plush.

Vit're-ous. Having the appearance of glass ; applied to a fluid in the cavity of the eyeball.

Vo-cal Cords. Two elastic bands in the windpipe; the essential parts of the organ of voice.

INDEX